The SomaVeda® Holistic Healing Bible

50 Systems of Indigenous Thai Yoga Therapy, Ayurvedic Healing, and Somatic Energy Balancing

Anthony B. James

The SomaVeda® Holistic Healing Bible: 50 Systems of Indigenous Thai Yoga Therapy, Ayurvedic Healing, and Somatic Energy Balancing

By Anthony B. James DNM(P), ND(T), MD(AM)

Ajahn and Master teacher of SomaVeda Integrated Traditional Therapies® :Indigenous, Traditional Thai Yoga & Ayurveda

Inquiries should be addressed to: Anthony B. James, DNM(P), ND, MD(AM)
Publisher: Meta Journal Press • 8491 Central Ave. Brooksville, FL 34613

(706) 358-8646, Email: nativeaic@gmail.com

Websites: Native American Indigenous Church: NAIC, Inc. NativeFireChurch.org

The Thai Yoga Center: ThaiYogaCenter.Com

American College of Natural Medicine: NAIC-Edu.org Natural Wellness Solutions Tribal Clinic: NaicTribalWellness.org

ISBN: 978-1-886338-52-4

Library of Congress Control No. # 2026912689

Printed in the U.S.A

Cover Illustration by Anthony B. James

Original art and photography by Anthony B. James Typography by Anthony B. James, Design art and original design by Anthony B. James SomaVeda® Integrated Traditional Therapies® is a Trademarked (US Patent Reg. No. 4,304,611-Registered Mar. 19, 2013 and Reg. No. 7,513,621 Renewal of Registration Spp. 24, 2024 Int. CL.: 44), proprietary system of religious therapeutics, holistic wellness, health, healing, way of life, Humanitarian Aid Service, based primarily on Thai Traditional Medicine (*Thai Ayurveda*), Thai Ayurveda (*Ryksaa Thaang Nuad Phaen Boran Thai*) and martial arts.

ISBN-13: 978-1-886338-52-4

53499

9 781886 338524

Dedication

To all my teachers and students who inspire me to reach deeper every day more than the last.

Introduction / Foreword

Welcome to the forefront of modern holistic healing. In a world where mainstream Western allopathic medicine often relies on managing symptoms and suppressing disease with chemicals, a profound need has emerged for true, root-cause resolution. *The SomaVeda® Holistic Healing Bible* answers this call by presenting a free-standing, whole-system of natural medicine that seamlessly bridges the ancient and the modern.

SomaVeda Integrated Traditional Therapies® is not merely a collection of techniques, nor is it commercial "massage therapy". **It is a comprehensive, functional medicine paradigm and a genuine form of alternative medicine.** Drawing upon the indigenous wisdom of Thai Ayurveda, classical Indian medicine, and spiritual native traditions, SomaVeda® treats the human body as a dynamic, interconnected matrix of physical, mental, and spiritual energy. It is holistic in every sense of the word, recognizing that the body, mind, and spirit cannot be isolated; their functions are interdependent and synergistic.

What makes this book revolutionary is its capacity to serve as a **complementary counterpart to mainstream Western medical systems** rather than an adversary. By integrating ancient energetic frameworks, such as the "*Tri-Dosha*", "*Chakras*", "*Thai Sen*" lines, and Native American Medicine concepts of wholeness and health as a spiritual understanding of health being an indication with "Mother Earth" and God, with cutting-edge 21st-century integrative science like the TOBIN Protocol, SomaVeda® offers unparalleled applications.

It offers practitioners the precise tools needed to combat complex modern illnesses, syndromes, and **"Biopathies,"** the physical rigidity and emotional distress caused by today's unprecedented environmental toxins, oxidative stress, and trauma that, in Ayurveda terms, are defined as "Dosha Imbalance" or a disordered relationship of "*tri-dosha*".

Whether you are a seasoned medical professional looking to integrate genuine holistic therapies into your existing practice or an individual seeking a deeply rewarding career in spiritually based, ethical, and moral holistic services, this book is your ultimate blueprint.

Through over 50 distinct therapeutic systems, ranging from dynamic, co-facilitated Hatha Yoga, Traditional Thai "*Nuad Boran*", and Ayurveda Pancha Karma/ Marma Chikitsa to the revolutionary Tool Assisted Energy Line Release (TAELR) protocol. SomaVeda® teaches you to facilitate profound healing for almost any condition.

Prepare to discover a path of healing defined by the "Four Divine States of Mind": Love, Compassion, Joy, and Equanimity. Step into a new paradigm where you can offer the world natural, non-invasive, and life-affirming care, returning true health sovereignty to your clients and yourself.

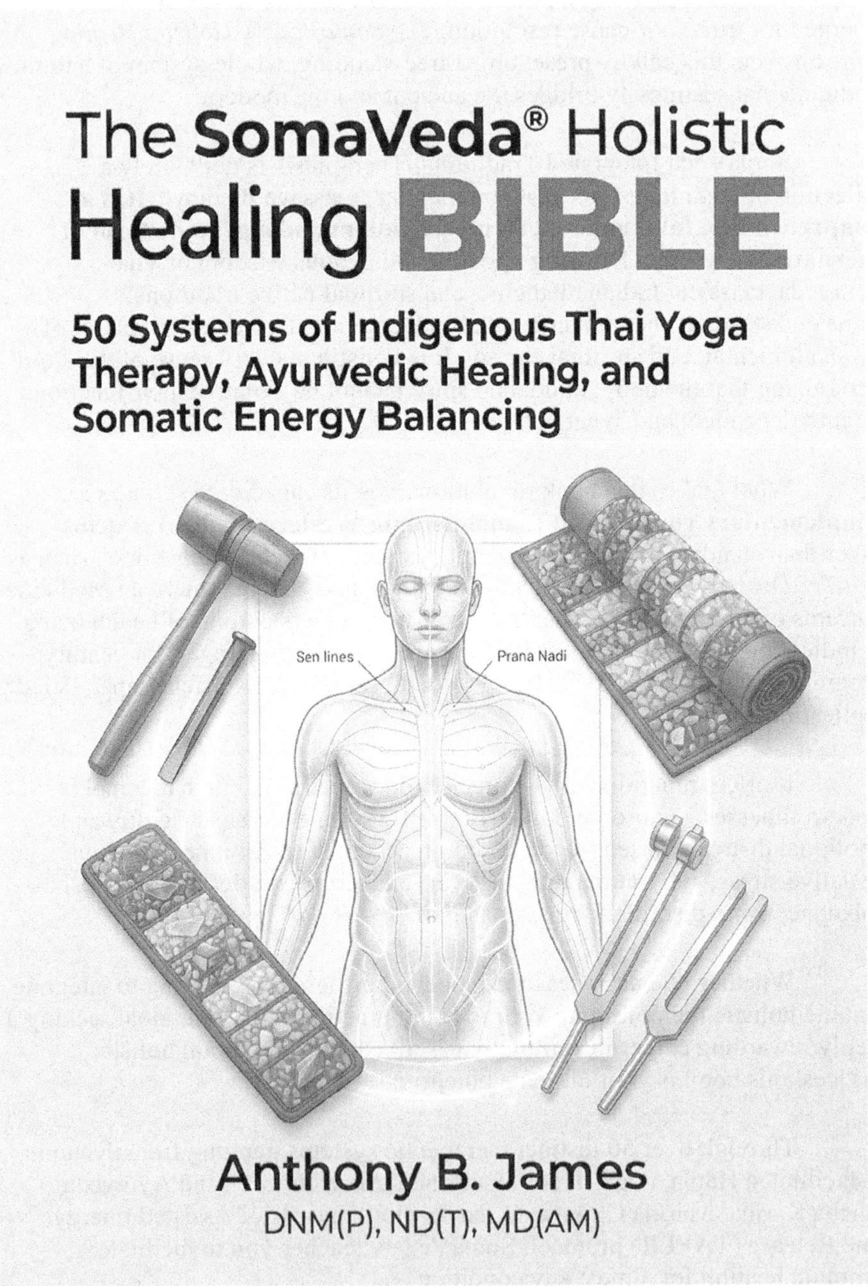

Table of Contents

What are SomaVeda Integrated Traditional Therapies®?

Also known as "SomaVeda®" Thai Yoga Therapy. It is based on the integration of indigenous, traditional, and spiritually based healing sciences and systems of both Eastern and Western origins. The ancient and modern systems that form the basis of SomaVeda® originate from several countries and cultures, including Thailand, India, China, Tibet, the Philippines, Indonesia, Malaysia, Japan, and the Americas.

The most important category of contribution to SomaVeda® is that of the Indigenous Traditional Thai Medicine (Ayurveda of Thailand) and Indigenous Traditional Thai Yoga and Medical Massage from the "*Buddhai Sawan*", "*Buntautuk*", "*Thai Phra Wat Chetuphon-Wat Po*", "*Anantasuk rongrian*" and "*Lek Chaiya Jap Sen Nuad*" traditional schools. In particular, the primary techniques are based on the Royal and Northern branches of Indigenous Traditional Thai Medicine (ITTM/TTM), as defined and registered by the Union of Thai Traditional Medicine Society (UTTS) and the Wat Po Association of Thai Traditional Medical Schools.

These various systems, forming subsets of practice in SomaVeda®, are initially taught in the strictest forms, as originally learned from those schools by Ajahn Dr. Anthony B. James. These systems form the technical basis for the SomaVeda® techniques. Additional influences of Traditional Chinese Medicine (TCM), Classical Indian Ayurveda, Western drugless Naturopathy (ANMA style traditional drugless Nature Cure), Christian Monastic Medicine (Medicine of Hope- SMOKH), Japanese Shiatsu (Sensei Toshiko Phipps, Sensei Kiku Miyasaki, Sensei Shizuto Yamamoto, and Sifu Dr. Doann T. Kaneko) and Indigenous Traditional Native American Medicine are the key therapies which are integrated into SomaVeda®. Thai Indigenous medicine has historically included the input and practical applications of healing found in the places where it was practiced.

We have seen traditional, energy-based systems, such as TCM, TTM, Homeopathy, Native American Medicines, and mainstream Western Medicine, including Allopathy, Osteopathy, and Psychology, long portrayed as opposed to one another. Although this has been largely true in the past, it is now possible for us to lay down our swords… the criticisms and competitive posturing we have been using to denigrate and compete, which will create the optimum environment for many types of healing experiences.

As we move away from a place where the definition of wellness and health is the "absence of disease", and to one that defines health as "a state of complete physical, mental [spiritual] and social well-being and not merely the absence of disease or infirmity. The definition seeks to include social and economic sectors within the scope of attaining health and reaffirms health as a human right" (WHO Alma-Ata Declaration 1978).

We will explore a model that portrays the human patient as a complete whole. Body, mind, and spirit cannot be taken or considered as separate, unrelated parts of us. Separating these three components is only a mental exercise, for in reality, they are one. There are variations in perspective, more or less evident as one looks at a person from different angles and prejudices. Their functions and existence overlap and are interdependent, synergistic, and sympathetic to a degree, as we only begin to suspect.

The body, the mind, and the spirit working together create the instrument by which our very soul is manifest and able to interact and to communicate with the material world and the universe of which we are a part. In indigenous, traditional medicine, humans are described as being "conduits" between the twin powers of the Celestial influences and energies of Heaven and the terrestrial influences and energies of the Earth. We are how the Heavens feel wet grass between the toes and how the earth sees the stars.

Native Americans say "Mitakoe Oyasin" (Lakota), "we are all relatives." This implies that we are living constituents of all life and are directly related to all life in some way.

It is only when we begin to see the energetic potential and its physical manifestations that we are "seeing" the real person. There is no such thing as a body apart from the energy and vitality that animates and communicates through it. The Tibetans say our body is "a perfected manifestation, a perfect luminosity" of our consciousness. Take a corpse, for example, no matter how intact or whole or complete we find it, it resembles a live person in merest form only. The corpse bears a superficial resemblance which diminishes immediately and continues to diminish until it returns to the earth from which it was initially borrowed.

We cannot isolate the various qualities and energies that human beings manifest from the physical body. We call these qualities "Life", and traditional healing medicines (religious therapeutics) have sought to define the nature of this Life force or vital essence as energies and qualities of sacred spirit.

The Vehicle of Life

In creating this new and vital way of health, we will focus on the body as a dynamic vehicle with qualities of life and spirit that together create a matrix of energy. This energy matrix encourages matter to coalesce in a particular way. The result of this coalescing of matter will be the manifestation of a human being with various attributes. What makes up the ***Stress Adaptive Human Biological Transformational Machine***?

Shen:
The spiritual essence of being (The Atman, The Soul). This is the fundamental or vital elixir that calls forth the creation of life, ultimately manifesting as men and women.

The Matrix Body:
Existing as a pure energy field. A field with characteristics common to electromagnetic energy, but of an as-yet-undefined frequency. This Matrix Body is the energetic framework that our visible body emulates. Properties of vibrations govern the matrix body, and as such, it has universal qualities exceeding the limitations of time and space as we commonly know them. Astrology, for example, is an attempt to reconcile the observance of these universal properties.

The construction of this Matrix Body has been better known and described in man's history than in present times. For example, in ancient Indian Sanskrit, the English word "Prayer" can be defined in as many as 64 different ways. The vocabulary to even describe sublime principles is lacking in the West. Perhaps to paraphrase Lao Tsu, from the "Dao De Jing" commonly called the "Tao", "language cannot encompass all that there is." However, we do have some information, and there have been clues left for us.

With these "clues" and traditional teachings, we use our own intuitions as the ancients did, as well as our modern intelligence, to reinvent and co-create the present understanding. We bring the "Science of Life" to the knowledge and awareness of mankind at a time when it is most needed.

Chi or Prana are the qualities most commonly associated with the Matrix Body. The medium, qualities, and elements associated with the manifestation of Chi and Prana constitute the energetic anatomy and physiology of Meridians, Sen, Prana Nadi, Chakra, Acupoints, Channels, vessels, Five Elements, Yin/Yang, and all such concepts.

The M.E.I.S. Body:
The Mental, Emotional, Instinctive, and Sexual body. The MEIS body is created through the interaction among the Matrix body, the Shen or spiritual essence, the Tangible Physical Body (TPB) (the sum of our material parts), and the reality of the environment in which the triad comes into existence.

What we know as a person's personality and psychology is generated here and reflected in the mirror of the ***Tangible Physical Body*** (TPB), also known as the Somatic Body. Beyond this, physical reality may also be imparted to or communicated through the MEIS body in various ways. The communication is eventually found reflected in each energetic body in turn.

By energetic bodies, there are basically two schemes that come to mind. The first is hierarchical and follows the general relationship of the Chakras and their correlations, progressing from lower to higher frequencies. Each body in turn is resonant and or in communication with a specific order or realm in the Ray of Creation. This theory posits that we are multidimensional beings composed of seven levels of energy, each vibrating at a distinct rate.

From lowest vibration to highest, the seven levels are from Physical to Spirit:

1. **The Physical/Etheric Level**
2. **The Emotional Level**
3. **The Lower Mental Level**
4. **The Astral Level**
5. **The Higher Mental Level**
6. **The Buddhic Level**
7. **The Spirit Level**

The second scheme of different energetic bodies is derived from classical Ayurveda. Theory of Koshas or Sheaths of consciousness. They are:

1. **Annamayi Kosha:** Sheath of Matter: The densest and purely physical body.
2. **Pranamayi Kosha:** Sheath of Vital Air: The body of breath and or Prana.
3. **Manomayi Kosha:** Sheath of Mind: The Cognitive, Intellectual body.
4. **Vijnanamayi Kosha:** Sheath of Knowledge: The Awareness/ Being body.
5. **Anandamayi Kosha:** Sheath of Bliss: The heart, spirit, and "Oneness" body.

The Somatic Body (TPB) is the subconscious mind.

The Somatic Body is the location of the personality and psychology of a person's mind. The Somatic body is the result of a process that begins with the Shen, Matrix, and MEIS bodies interacting with the closest stellar bodies we know of: the Sun, Moon, and Earth. On a relative scale of vibrational frequency, the Somatic body is the lowest and slowest of all the various bodies.

This idea also brings to bear the concept of "We are Many". We call the composite the "Great" body or "*Somata Magnifica*". We, in fact, are composed of many overlapping representations of energy, material, and frequency, which compose the form "I" or "Us". This is appropriate, from the beginning of creation, our Great Body has been transforming higher vibrations of one order to lower and transmuting lower vibrations of one order to a higher.

The TPB is the repository and storage bank for the MEIS body. It is also a material mirror, or tangible image, of MEIS's organization. As such, we say the TPB is the subconscious mind. It is where the personality constructs and psychology reside.

The construction of the TPB is well understood and documented in the biological sciences and well known through the study of anatomy and physiology of Western medical science. However, no current Anatomy & Physiology text describes the functions and components of the human body in relation to its more esoteric, energetic aspects.

These are the aspects and qualities that more or less relate to the MEIS body, the Matrix body, and the Shen, Astral, spirit, or essence being of a person. No clear descriptions of functions will be considered complete until all of these relationships are addressed individually and holistically. The need is to examine the role of each component, seeking additional clues about their place and role in the ray of creation. Studying the Enneagram as described in the book "Korosot Astrology" (Anthony B. James) and/or the literature on Fourth Way psychology (Gurdjieff, Ouspensky, Bennett, Nicole, etc.) may provide a resource for understanding many of the processes and functions of the human organism.

SomaVeda® is a way of life rooted in great compassion for the suffering of human beings and the belief that, through a deeper understanding of ourselves, we might, in the end, be of greater value. SomaVeda® is a system of religious therapeutics in the broadest sense of the word and is not meant to be taken strictly as physical rehabilitation.

SomaVeda® borrows and integrates concepts and applications from the world's great spiritual and sacred traditions of health and healing, such as Indigenous Classical Indian Ayurveda, Traditional Chinese Medicine, Indigenous Traditional Thai Medicine, Native American, and Western Monastic Naturopathy (Nature Cure). There is no restriction or limitation to the concept of recovering ground or function that has been lost. We explore breaking the common limitations and boundaries on our existence through the medium of healing work. We come before the seemingly insurmountable walls of our paradigms regarding life, health, consciousness, energy, and capacity with a conscious perspective. The reason why rehabilitation of disability, injury, or trauma is so complex is that we do not understand what our normal is. Our views of ourselves are fragmented at best.

How can a science or an art of health truly hope to reestablish harmony, balance, and function when these concepts are not understood correctly, if at all? Western science is only now beginning to admit the possibility that there might be other, less tangible factors in a person's physical health beyond their specific pathologies! This has been understood, and there is evidence of this understanding since time immemorial in sacred and or religious societies. It is only in the current age of man that this understanding is not generally expressed.

The very idea of a person's energetic makeup should not be esoteric. There exist many different likely avenues that are capable of producing, transferring, carrying, or transporting the various forms of energy ascribed to the body.

For example, ancient traditions refer to many simultaneous, overlapping, and integrated bodies. The ancient Hindu Vedic scriptures, for example, referred to "350,000" Prana Nadi four thousand years ago. The people of Thailand and the surrounding areas, in their traditional scriptures (sacred texts or Codices), relate how 72,000 lines of energy within the body, referred to as Sen (Prana Nadi), were condensed into a network of 10 primary lines. Ancient Chinese culture produced documents and teachings that were used for thousands of years and served a similar function. They identified 12 primary channels and 2 extraordinary vessels, known as meridians. They also went further with theories that incorporated Transverse Subcutaneous Muscle channels (fascia), muscle channels, and connecting vessels. All of these things attempt to reconcile direct observation of the body's "nonphysical" phenomenon.

In one sense, as Westerners, we have not seen the forest for the trees. Western researchers have been trying for many years to locate a set of nerves or other mechanisms related to, or similar to, what is described as Meridians, Nadi, Sen, etc. One such researcher was Dr. Robert O.

Becker, MD. Former head of research for the Veterans Administration, USA.

He postulated and actually demonstrated the existence of what he called a DC Potential Field or Morphogenic Field, which would allow for the possibility of acupuncture as a valid concept, even from the point of view of Western science. He postulated that this field operates as a control system through semiconduction. A phenomenon that is only now being researched and understood in relation to its application to living organisms.

Other researchers have brought to bear the magnetic field theories, demonstrating the body's ability to internally produce electric fields, magnetic fields, and EMF (Electromotive Force- Thermal). Even variations of fields of varying intensity and polarity relative to specific organs! Western Science, which has been so quick to criticize traditional theories and methodologies based upon them, is itself only in the last few years developing technologies and understandings to substantiate what the traditional cultures have known and experienced for thousands of years. These ancient cultures developed these understandings, not using sophisticated technologies, but their abilities of intuition and observation!

We are in a unique position in that, at present, probably for the first time in the history of mankind, we have access to both the traditional concepts, understandings, and methodologies and the modern, Western scientific understanding and view of things. Not to mention that we at the same time live in the most precarious time relating to the variety and severity of health issues altogether. The watchwords and concepts for SomaVeda® are respect for traditional concepts and lineage, complementation, integration, application, mastery, community, puja, and compassion.

SomaVeda® Thai Yoga represents a holistic, comprehensive approach to addressing the complex issue of Biopathy, or disturbance to the proper functioning of the stress-adaptive human biologic transformational machine, or person.

What is Indigenous Traditional Thai Yoga?

Since the basis of SomaVeda® Integrated Traditional Therapies® is Indigenous Traditional Thai Medicine (ITTM), Thai Yoga, or Traditional Thai Massage, let's answer the question "What is Thai Yoga?"

ITTM is an ancient, indigenous, traditional, spiritually based system of healing, Chirothesia, and Somatic therapy in which the healer, practitioner,
therapist, doctor, or family member (provider) literally becomes the extension of sacred, divine intention, manifestation, and expression. The provider becomes the embodiment of the sacred spirit of healing. It is a direct, literal, practical expression of compassion and loving-kindness, reducing suffering, enhancing life, and bringing health, wellness, and happiness to all who are touched by it. ITTM is as beneficial to all providers in all respects as it is to the receiver.

ITTM and/or Traditional Thai Massage represent the most authentic visions of Indigenous Traditional Thai Medicine, Thai Culture, and related healing arts that the Thai people have always considered sacred. Our Instructors are directly authorized teachers, representatives, and traditional lineage holders in several different traditional Buddhist schools:
1) Buddhai Sawan Institute Ayutthaya and Nongkam (famous for martial and healing arts for 900 years!),
2) Phra Wat Chetuphon (Buddhist Temple, Wat Po Traditional Thai Medical School...One of the oldest schools of traditional arts),
3) "*Wat Raja-Orasarem*" in Korat province,
4) Buntautuk Hill tribes Northern Provincial Hospital and Training Institute, also known as "The Old Medicine Hospital of *Shivago Komarpai*".
5) ITM (International Thai Massage, Chiangmai),
6) Mama Lek Chaiya (Jap Sen Nuad, Wat Suan Dok Style, Chiangmai)
7) The Foundation for the Blind, Buddhist Temple "*Wat Wianglock.*"
8) "*Wangklaikangwon*" Industrial Community & Educational College program sponsored by HM. King Bhumibol, *Anantasuk* Thai Massage,
9) The UTTS or Union of Thai Traditional Medicine Society
10) As well as several other significant lineages, teachers, and Grand Masters.

According to Vichai Chokevivat, M.D., M.P.H, Department for the Development of Thai Traditional and Alternative Medicine, Ministry of Public Health, Thailand [27]

"TTM is regarded as comprising the traditional philosophies, bodies of knowledge, and modes of practice to care for the health of Thai people that are congruent with Thai culture and way of life and based on the principles of Buddhism. TTM uses various forms of practice that complement each other, i.e., medicine, pharmacy, massage (Chirothesia), midwifery and maternal and child health care, Buddhist rites and meditation, as well as other rituals based on belief in supernatural power or the power of the universe. TTM is a holistic and natural approach to health care that is derived from Buddhist beliefs, the observation of and respect for nature, and the wisdom of Thai ancestors."

In addition, traditional knowledge of TTM was also built through the processes of "selection", "adoption", "adaptation", and "utilization" of traditional medicine of some countries with which Thailand had contact in the past, e.g., India, Malaysia, Japan, China, and the Philippines, to suit the Thai way of life.

One thing you can say about our tradition is that many of the technical practices are literally carved in stone! Many visitors to Thailand will be familiar with the famous "*Epigraphies of King Rama*" located on the grounds of Wat Po in Bangkok. Wat Po has become one of the most visited religious sites in Thailand. It is revered by Thai and foreign tourists alike, but for different reasons.

In addition to the famous "*Epigraphies of King Rama*" (Carved stone medical texts) located at "*Wat Po*" and "*Wat Raja-Orasarem*" (Built by King Rama III: in the Thai/ Chinese style called "The Royal Favorable Art" style), there are also gunite statues of Thai Reishi Yogis practicing the various Asana or traditional Yoga postures - The Thai variation of Hatha Yoga or self-treatment. In the past, there were more than 100 of these interesting figures scattered about the courtyards of Wat Po. However, over the years, many were damaged or deteriorated by weathering and have been retired for preservation. The Yoga practices of the ancient Thai Reishi (Sacred Mystics, hermits, and Ayurveda practitioners) are referred to as "Reusi Dottan".

In Thailand's past, people came to temples for just about everything, from medical care to education. Anyone could come to the temple for food, shelter, medical care, or spiritual healing. ITTM (Traditional Thai Medicine/Traditional Thai Massage) contributed to the emotional, physical, and spiritual well-being of the ancient Thais, and it continues to do so today.

Most importantly, the Buddhist medicine associated and derived from the famous Buddhist Saint "*Shivago Khumarbaaca*" (Jivaka). In the

US, traditional lineage and teaching are primarily passed on via the educational programs of the Thai Yoga Center in Brooksville, FL. Additionally, we recognize any schools formally licensed as legal Traditional Thai Yoga and/or Thai Massage schools by the Royal Thai Ministries of Health and Education, whether listed or not!

The type of Thai traditional therapy that most people will be directly exposed to is "*ráksãa thaang nûat phaen boran thai*" ("*Marma Chikitsa*" ancient healing marma and yoga therapy treatment). This is more commonly known as the Nuad Thai or Nuad Boran styles of ITTM therapy, or the spiritual massage (Chirothesia/*Marma Chikitsa*), the healing work of Thailand.

Please note, for clarity, that although in common English we use the word "massage," we do not mean it in the same context as the typical Western usage. In the West, "Massage" is often used as a synonym for a "Rub Down" for money and primarily refers to systems derived from Swedish Massage and Massage Therapy. "Thai Yoga and or Thai Massage" (*Phaen Boran Ráksãa Thaang Nûat)* is completely unrelated! It is a religious therapeutic healing art derived from Theraveda Buddhism, Buddhist medicine, Classical Indian and Tibetan Ayurveda, and Yoga Vedanta.

It is not required that one become a religious practitioner to practice this healing art; however, just because non-religious persons and/or those with no defined faith practice this healing method does not make it non-spiritual or non-sacred! Just because a non-religious person takes some techniques away from the tradition to use in their commercial practice does not make this indigenous traditional healing art less of a system of religious therapeutics.

It would be more accurate to call this medicine either by its traditional names or "Ancient, Anachronistic or Old Thai Way of Healing with The Hands", so long as the slang term "Thai Massage" is in use, there will be understandable confusion.

Primary Outcomes

The primary outcomes associated with the practice of ITTM are called "*ProMiiWihan Sii*" or Four Divine, or Boundless States of mind without limitation. They are Love, Compassion, Joy, and Equanimity. As long as these four qualities are communicated, transmitted, and exemplified during a session, we say it was good and successful.

For this reason, it is possible to have an ITTM session with little or even no actual touching! In addition to the four divine states of mind, we practice and perform Puja (Prayer/ ritual healing). PUJA is a multi-step protocol first to acknowledge the sacred space shared by the client and healer, and to honor and acknowledge the Bodhisattvas and progenitors of our way and teaching. PUJA directs one to "*Generate the Boddichitta,*" or perfected mental processes of enlightened beings, through the recitation of the "Om Namo Shivago" mantra, the Metta Sutra, or similar. Invoking and inviting the essences and energies of love and healing to move within the body of ourselves and our client, and listening to sacred attunements.

This prayerful and thoughtful meditation and attuning to various energies, and petitioning of sacred and symbolic metaphors of deity, ancient guides, the literal flesh-and-blood examples for our modern practice, the role models, provide the basis for all further communication and expression of thoughtful ideals. Puja practice is a functional practice of "giving credit, where credit is due, reminding us also that we did not invent this beautiful work of medicine and healing. We inherited it. It is a source of humility and confidence to see how what we are practicing was proven in the past, carried forward to our generation, and now delivers the same high level of functionality and positive outcomes as before.

SomaVeda® Thai Yoga has its own Noble Eightfold Path.

YAMAS: Good Way of Life (Internal: Not expressing negativity. Think good thoughts. Generate BoddhiChitta.)

NIYAMA: Good Way of Life (External: Bring love into the world. Practice external considerations: Use of prayers and chants (Mantra), study, and charity. Do good things.

ASANA: Practical Exercise (For yourself and others), SomaVeda®, Martial Arts, Hatha Yoga, Invest in personal development for yourself and others. Develop yourself and others. Keep yourself as healthy as possible.

PRANAYAMA: Breath Science (Facilitation of 5 Pranas), Bandhas (Locks and Windgates), Mudras, and Mantra (Focus and direct energy). Cultivate awareness of breath and Intention. Breathe on purpose! Breath is the vital life force, the essence of life and consciousness given to us by God and the Great Spirit.

WAI KHRUU: (Puja) Paying Respect to the Teachers (Pratyahara). Give credit where credit is due. Make acknowledgment a way of life,

SAMATHA: Shamatha, Dharana (Calm Abiding Meditation). Don't Panic! Wait, and things will change.

VIPASSANA: Dhyana (Insight Meditation). Three kinds of meditations: Walking, Sitting, and sharing SomaVeda® ®. Find your real abiding mind in thought, action, and deed.

PROMIIWIHAN SII:

Four Divine States of Mind (Love, Compassion, Joy, and Equanimity) Samadhi. Make love and four divine states of mind your basic motivation... Work toward love, stay with it, come from that place.

Secondary Outcomes

The secondary outcomes, of lesser importance, may or may not share characteristics with many forms of Western massage.

such as effleurage (stroking and kneading the muscles), non-ballistic manual facilitation into Yoga postures (manipulating or moving/ aligning osseous or skeletal parts) and pressure point (Marma Chikitsa) or acupressure style technique (applying deep, consistent pressure to specific nerves, tendons, or ligaments and acupoints traditionally referred to as Marma/ Lom) to balance the functions of the four body elements called "*thâat tháng sìi*" (*Lom, Fai Din, Naam*).

Thai Yoga incorporates elements of energetic and Prana assessment, mindfulness, gentle rocking, Asana positional release, deep stretching, focused breathing or *PranaYama*, Chakra balancing, Prana Nadi or Sen line balancing, and rhythmic compression to restore oneness with God and Spirit, creating a singular healing experience.

However, as we said previously, any applications of physical pressure are intended mainly to convey the Primary intentions of "*ProMiiwihan Sii*" to balance and harmonize the "Thaat Thang Sii" or four elements and Tri-dosha (also referred to as Three Winds, Humors, and or Energetically based Body Types). Much like the physical contact of a hug can convey care, consideration, and love, physical contact is highly sophisticated.

The four Thai Primary Ayurvedic Elements are: Earth (Din-solid parts of the body, including nerves, skeleton, muscles, blood vessels, tendons, and ligaments); Water (*Náam*-blood and bodily secretions); Fire (Fai-digestion and metabolism); and Air (Lom-respiration, and circulation). Borrowing from India's Ayurvedic tradition, some practitioners employ Pali-Sanskrit terms for the four bodily elements: "*pathavidhatu, apodhatu, tecodhatu, and vayodhatu*". The book "Lines, Wheels, Points and Specific Remedies" covers this theory in detail.
ITTM is Yoga.

Let me emphasize, ITTM is not LIKE Yoga, it IS Yoga!

From the Ayutthaya period until early this century, the Thai government's Department of Health included an official Ayurveda Nuad (Marma Chikitsa/ massage) division (*phanâek mãw nûat*). Under the influence of international medicine and modern hospital development, responsibility for the national propagation/maintenance of Indigenous Traditional Thai Ayurveda was eventually transferred to Phra Wat Chetaphon (Wat Pho) in Bangkok, where it remains today. Traditional Yoga therapy has persisted primarily in the provinces, however, and has recently enjoyed a resurgence of popularity throughout the country. The Wat Po system is divided into two completely separate and distinctive categories:

A) the tourist massage pavilion and Tourist massage school (*Rongrian Sala Thaang Nuad*)

B) the School for Traditional Medicine for training and certification of *Maw Nuad* (also *Moh Nuad*) (Traditional Doctors of Indigenous Traditional Thai Medicine and Ayurveda).

There are huge differences in the terms and quality of training. For example, a tourist may receive an introductory massage certificate in as little as 10 days, whereas the full Maw Nuad program is 12 to 14 semesters or four full years! In the States, we have many different levels of recognition for Certified ITTM/Traditional Thai Massage Practitioners.

The SomaVeda® Thai Yoga-based Associate of Sacred Arts (ASA) program is a two-year program that qualifies graduates to sit for the Traditional Naturopathic National Boards. A traditional Western Naturopath is considered by many to be the top of the holistic pyramid. We now have an established program to educate Traditional Naturopaths (Doctor of Sacred Natural Medicine) in the traditional healing methods of Thai Yoga!

In northern Thailand, which is closer to mainland China, you see more Chinese-, Laotian-, Mon-, and Khmer-influenced methods and techniques. For example, a well-known Teacher and practitioner in Chiang Mai, Mama Lek Chaiya and her family teach what is called "*nûat jàp sên*" (nerve-touch massage- "*Wat Suandok*" method), a Chinese-style massage technique that works with the body's nerve meridians, much like acupuncture.

Some of the plucking techniques are reminiscent of Chinese Tuina and can be quite unpleasant. However, the ultimate aim of balancing the Chi takes precedence over comfort! Please note: Mama Lek's practice was deeply spiritual and therapeutic in every way. She never touched a person or taught a class that was not from start to finish based on the spiritual expression of her religious beliefs. Every class and session began and ended with Puja… no exceptions. Her practice was a true example of a spiritual emphasis over techniques, a quality shared by Northern practitioners in general.

Within the Traditional Thai medical context, a Marma/ Lom therapist (*mãw nûat*, literally, 'Ayurveda massage doctor') usually applies ITTM together with pharmacological (herbal) and/or psycho-spiritual treatments as prescribed for a specific problem or specific imbalance of the Dosha or winds and humors of the body, mind, and spirit. It is becoming increasingly common for many Thais to use traditional massage for relaxation and disease prevention, rather than for a specific medical problem. However, once you leave the big city and move into the country, you begin to see greater reliance on the application as an energy-based medicine.

ITTM, Thai Yoga, and/or Traditional Thai Massage are not the same as "Massage, Massage Therapy," and/or "bodywork" as commonly defined in so-called "Massage Laws." The term "Thai Massage" is Western slang, mostly promoted by tourists in Thailand. Although the term is now common, it is still misunderstood and misused by the uninformed and/or misinformed. It is easy to be confused as similar words are used, such as "Massage", but legally there are distinctions and differences in definitions... In law, specific words may have different meanings and weights than those same words commonly associated by ordinary "Non-legal" or in lay speech/ speak.

For example, the definitions of "massage " and Massage Therapy" are based on the general practice known as "Swedish massage". So-called "Swedish Massage" is new (less than 100 years), Western (Europe and America) and defined legally as "the application of a system of structured touch, pressure, movement and holding to the soft tis- sues of the human body to affect the health and well-being of the client positively. The practice includes the external application of water, heat, cold, lubricants, salt scrubs, and other topical preparations and devices that mimic or enhance the actions of the hands."

ITTM, Traditional Thai Yoga, and/or Traditional Thai Massage sound a bit similar at first glance; however, the preceding definition does not mention that ITTM, Traditional Thai Yoga, and/or Thai Massage is a system of movement education (Yoga and co-facilitated Yoga). It is based entirely on principles of energy balancing (*Thai Sen, Tri-Dosha, Lom, Chakra*, etc.), and the actual touching, contact, or soft-tissue manipulation is incidental to, and not the central aim of, the practice!

As described above, the primary outcomes associated with the practice are called "*ProMiiWihan Sii*" or Four Divine, Boundless, or States of mind without limitation. They are Love, Compassion, Joy, and Equanimity. As long as these four qualities are transmitted and exemplified during a session, we say it was good and successful. For this reason, it is possible to have an ITTM session with little or even no actual touching! However, touching is good! ITTM incorporates elements of mindfulness, gentle rocking, deep stretching, rhythmic compression, and focus to create a singular healing experience.

This work brings fundamental elements and energy into harmony, creating wholeness of mind, body, and spirit. SomaVeda® Thai Yoga/Traditional Thai Massage is a spiritually based, religious, therapeutic, somatic technique and profession, a modality with standards originally established in the ancient Buddhist holistic centers and temples of Asia and Southeast Asia thousands of years ago. It has an established code of ethics, first coined by our ancient founder, "*Jivaka Kumarbhacca,*" derived from the Buddha Dharma and other similar or related sources. There is an established educational criterion for education and professional practice for services which are unrelated to and not intended to be implied as being "Massage " or "Massage therapy".

There are quite a few different traditional "schools" of ITTM. They range from the big university-driven or supported programs in Bangkok to the "Family"- style oral and traditional lineages of the Northern Hill Tribes, such as the Karen, Lisu, Lahu, and Akha. The influence of indigenous Hill Tribe sacred traditional medicine is a growing factor in the modern expression of ITTM, especially in northern Thailand.

The most famous traditional school in the North is The Buntautuk Northern Hill Tribes Medical Hospital, or "The Old Medicine Hospital" as it is more commonly called. Under the auspices of Grand Master Aajan Sintorn Chaichagun (Who Transitioned in November 2005), it has become a national and international phenomenon. Teaching various levels of programs to Thai and Falang (foreigners) alike, Aajan Pha Khru Sintorn was also famous for his daily recitation of the Pali Om Namo Shivago mantra, a prayer, and an invocation for blessings. Every day, twice a day, he would lead the entire community in this rhythmic and beautiful traditional mantra for healing. In the north, they say you don't know Traditional Thai Massage until you know this mantra!

Today, the Wat Po Association of Traditional Doctors, members' schools, and Ajahns (Master Instructors) are bringing this work into the modern world. Famous schools and their headmasters, such as Anantasuk Rongrian under Ajahn Nantipa Anantasuk, work with the King's *Rajaprajanugroh* projects to fully document traditional medicine to preserve this rich heritage.

In the US today, the traditional lineages that are vital to the SOMAVED® Thai Yoga and Traditional Thai Massage are passed on via the NAIC (American College of Natural Medicine) and the Thai Yoga Center in Brooksville, Florida, through the Mastery and teaching of Ajahn Dr. Anthony B. James.

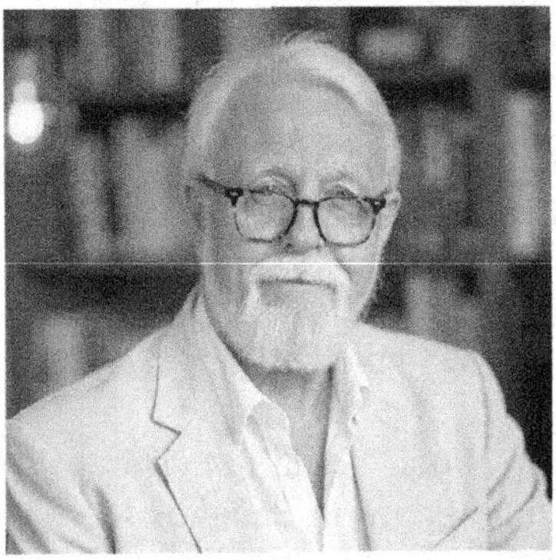

Ajahn James wrote and published the very first book in English, published in the US on Traditional Thai Yoga "Nuat Thai Traditional Thai Medical Massage", Meta Journal Press, Atlanta, Georgia, 1983: ISBN 1-886338-03-5.

Ajahn James demonstrates a SomaVeda® Indigenous Traditional Thai Yoga side lying position in Pang Lang village, Thailand: November 2009

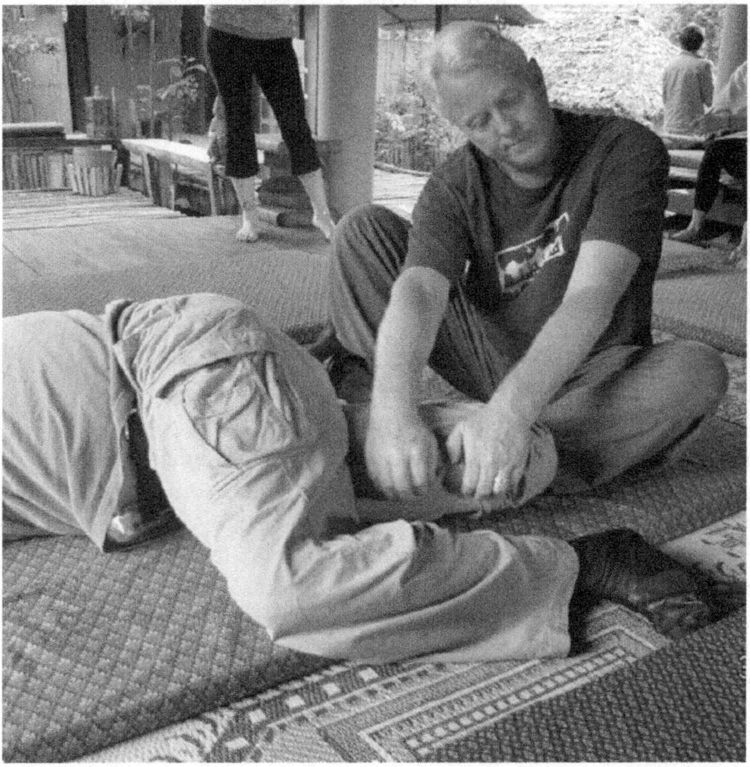

With 42+ years of extensive devotion, practice, and research, he brings several different and complementary traditional lineages to life. Additional credit must be given to the many teachers and instructors who have trained with Ajahn James over the years, as well as to the more than 20,000 students from over 32 countries who have completed training either directly facilitated by Ajahn or sponsored by him or one of his recognized SomaVeda®-certified teachers.

To learn more about the Thai Yoga Center and SomaVeda® Integrated Traditional Therapies®, visit https://ThaiYogaCenter.com.

What is Biopathy?

Biopathy is a contracture of the organism's Matrix and the TPB, emphasizing dominance of sympathetic nervous action and activity, i.e., "Sympatheticotonia".

What are the symptoms of Biopathy?

Psyche Symptoms are negative fear, phobia, anxiety, and general loss of conscious control of mental and emotional control in a spiral of deterioration.

a. Concentric movement and rigidity of physical and or postural attitude

b. Stiffness, Inflexibility of mind and mental process.

c. Reflexive conditioning and progressive submission to negative and increasingly negative thoughts and thought patterns.

d. Development of armoring and conditioned localized spasm forming both local areas of rigidity and corporately generalized loss of functions and circulation of life force, Prana, Chi, Orgone, as well as actual circulation of vital substances of the body i.e. fluids, secretions, oxygen, lymphatic and a corresponding increase in edema, stagnation and proportional atrophy of first local area tissue, then general deterioration of the entire system.

e. Energetically, this may be evidenced by imbalance and discord in the Matrix or energetic body, seen as discord in Dosha, Chakra, Sen, Nadi, Lom, and Marma. Hyper and or hypo sensitivity of Lom, acupoints, marma and lines, nadi and Sen. Restrictions and inability to assume asana and distortions of asana in practice, as well as reduced ability to perform common and ordinary movements and tasks of life. Efforts to do just about anything within the normal course of life would be or seem to be more difficult. This difficulty could be spiritual, mental, emotional, or physical. This difficulty might or might not be accompanied by pain.

f. Symptoms can also be combined in the sense of the bio-emotional, bio-physical, and bio-psychic. Bio-energetic and bio-sexual manifestations may occur in either sequence or all at once in varying degrees.

How does SomaVeda® address Biopathy?

SomaVeda® Technical Procedures:

1) Systematic decompression of the skeleton by use of co-facilitated Hatha Yoga postures. It is a system of general release and decompression of the entire system.

Following the principle of "The greatest potential for gain or loss of energy in the body's energy lines occurs in or at the joints or nexus of

osseous or bony structures in the body", all articulatory processes of the body are decompressed. Joint compression is identified and reduced as much as possible.
IMPORTANT: Additionally, it avoids counter-contracture or resistance to the decompression technique and methodology by using a non-ballistic, passive, assisted, or facilitated range of motion and compression.

2) Systematic decongestion. It reduces both apparent and hidden inflammation through broad, deep compression and targeted pressure on identifiable target regions of inflammation. Focus is on Sen Lines, Lom/Marma, Meridians, TSM, etc., using a wide variety of appropriate techniques and protocols.

3) Reduction of both apparent and hidden inflammations, edema, and all unusual or pathologic swellings, and areas of fluid retention with nonspecific general release techniques such as holding, inversions, rocking, coupled with pranayama. Inflammation is considered a sign of stagnation in attitude and energy, as well as of fluid.

4) Assess or check, target, treat, or focus and release all observed restrictions in all seven "Bridge Zones". Bridge zones are Dai Mo, or circular rings of both meridian and Chakra energy, in the sense of transverse meridians or "belt channels" that relate to specific Chakra influences. These Chakra Bridge Zones may also correlate with neuralgic dermal zones. They are rings of influence circumnavigating the round torso, neck, and head with importance on all of the "bodies". (Matrix, Kosha, M.E.I.S., TPB, etc.)

The Seven Chakra Bridge Zones are:

- Crown (Chakra Seven)
- Ocular (Chakra Six)
- Mandible (Chakra Five)
- Throat (Chakra Five)
- Chest/ Breast (Chakra Four)
- Diaphragm (Chakra Three)
- Abdomen (Chakra Two)
- Pelvic (Chakra One)

Since all healthy processes depend on the exchange of Prana, Air, Vital Life Force, Chi, Ki, Orgone, Mana, etc., SomaVeda® Thai Yoga Therapy promotes breath and consciousness of breath throughout. Focuses the breath on any obvious stagnant or "Stuck" areas and coaches and directs the breathing to support expressive movement in all zones in turn. This SomaVeda® Zone therapy is like a combination lock. Begin with Zone One, release it before moving on to Zone Seven.

5) Target with integration techniques in all physical areas where specific negative emotions are evident. i.e., tapping and affirmation (SomaVeda® BET/EFT).

6) Use Tapping (SomaVeda® BET/ EFT) for all negative emotional references: fear, phobia, neurosis, anxiety, compulsion, psychosis, and "Manias" as well as persistent pain of any kind. We believe that "The cause of all negative emotion is a disruption of the body's energy system". Furthermore, there is a component of negative emotion either as a fundamental or original cause or as a supporting negative influence and/ or modifier in all chronic and or debilitating illnesses and discomforts.

No treatment can be considered complete unless, at some point, negative emotional patterns, their symptoms, and the causative energy disruptions that underlie them are addressed in depth. The practitioner should also consider using or emphasizing tapping for any pain or sensitivities too severe for manual contact.

7) Allow and encourage the client to engage in free association, expression of feelings, and imagery, especially any that focuses on or targets restricted areas or patterns of contraction and/or inhibition. Guided meditation and rituals/ceremonies, such as the sweat lodge and drumming, can be used to enhance this expression and association.

8) Use noninvasive external applications of helpful modalities that support decongestion, reduce inflammation and spasm, increase circulation, and promote general relaxation of tension.

9) Use of resistance work and/or co-facilitation to bring or increase awareness of any areas where synesthesia or lack of communication is apparent.

10) Use of detoxification as appropriate, to reduce or to remove and diminish the effects of stored toxins and or allergens in the body. Pancha Karma regimens are indicated in these cases. Pancha Karma stimulates the immune system and reduces the inhibitory effect of the toxins in the body. This reduces the inflammatory process that is supported or even caused by toxins stored in the tissues. Herbal detox, far-infrared sauna, light therapies, and chelation may be good adjuncts to treatment.

11) With corrective nutrition or diet and promotion of a healthy eating lifestyle, by emphasizing a plant-based diet as appropriate for body type and or Dosha imbalance.

12) Specific use of physical, mental, emotional, and or spiritual (psychic) techniques of any kind to bring about, correct, or restore high-functioning equilibrium to the client. No matter which methods or combinations of methods, tools, and adjuncts are selected, they must remain essentially non-drug-based, non-surgical, natural, holistic, non-harmful, and non-injurious to both client and healer.

Regardless of the technical approach selected as most appropriate for the client, the SomaVeda® practitioner performs the healing service as an expression of love, care, consideration, and compassion as a religious observance and ministry. It is the sacerdotal or sacred duty of those in our community authorized and or ordained to literally become the hands of God, of the Great Spirit (Chirothesia).

This work is and always has been a religious therapy, a system of religious therapeutics. The fact that certain aspects have been taken out of the sacred tradition's context to make money or for commercial or political gain (e.g., Tourist Massage/"Massage Therapy") does not diminish the value of the full expression of ITTM for healing. In the US, we must especially keep in mind that just because we, indigenous, traditional Native, and/or spirit-based Medicine Persons, allow "Massage Therapists" to attend training does not in any way change the meaning, value, intention, sacredness, and indigenous traditional religious therapeutic medicine practice we observe.

Designing a SomaVeda® Indigenous Thai Yoga session.

Please note: SomaVeda® Religious Therapeutics (ITTM) and healing services, counseling, and/or therapies are performed by NAIC Tribal Org. authorized ministers/practitioners exclusively for other NAIC members. Any services performed by non-members and or on non-members are not protected under NAIC.

All Sessions and therapeutic day protocols begin and end with Puja, a five-step process that creates sacred space, prays for the client's well-being and healing, and involves listening. The sessions themselves are a form of religious therapy, exchanging love and compassion with the intention of creating a safe and trustworthy space for healing and the cure of disease.

Step 1: Assessment - Conduct a differential assessment to identify primary and secondary complaints, as well as any apparent issues. This assessment also determines if there are any extenuating factors or circumstances, such as toxic exposure, allergens, mental, emotional, or spiritual issues, or poor nutrition.

Step 2: Determining appropriate treatment application and strategy. What to do now or first, second, etc.

Step 3: Do the therapeutic day treatment program and apply the strategies.

Step 4: Reassess and measure responses and outcomes.
Step 5: Adjust or refine applications and procedures as the client adapts and responds.

Step 6: Coach and apply SomaVeda® BET/ EFT protocol for releasing and balancing the imbalances and conditions either caused by or supported by chronic negative emotional patterns.

Step 7: Consider strategies for maintenance and long-term monitoring, as needed.

Step 8: Complete the therapeutic process when either successful outcomes manifest, or the homeodynamic status and return to wellness and greater health and functionality are sustainable.

Everything that's alive moves!

Movement and motility are signs of life. As one surveys the body and the person in general, one observes what is simply not moving or motile compared with the surrounding structures, tissues, and functions. The function of everything in the person is to participate and support either contraction or expansion.

This contraction and expansion alternately represent the organic engines of the life process. There are no completely fixed or rigid structures in the body, even those considered "rigid," such as osseous tissues or bones. Even bones and other skeletal components in a healthy state are alive, malleable, flexible, and permeable. They are in a state of continuous expansion and contraction in all dimensions, reacting and adapting to both internal pressure and circulation, as well as external pressure on the surface.

Every Bone is a complete cosmos, an entity living a life of its own, unique and peculiar to its allocation of service in the body. This bone, however, shares its rhythm of life and function with the organic community of its environment within the body proper and responds and adapts to internal and external pressures and influences originating from said body proper.

The bones are integral to the functioning immune system, as the marrow, or the "hollow" center of the bones, is the origin of antibody production and T-cell production. We know without doubt that there is a connection between the immune system and the emotions. This leads us to the following statement: Emotions affect immune functions, which in turn affect osseous function, which subsequently affects immune functions, which ultimately affect emotions.

We also have reason to believe that the emotional state at any given moment in time, such as depression, resignation, anxiety, etc., can be reflective of the immune system's actions and status, suppressed or overly excited, as an example.

Again, osseous function and state can impact the immune system, which in turn can affect or be reflected in emotions. On the flip side, we see how emotions, chronic states of extreme or debilitating emotions, can depress the immune system.

That these strong negative, persistent emotional states can literally cause the body's healing functions of maintenance, defense, and growth to shut down indicates a two-way system of influence and dynamic interaction. A healthy, mobile, dynamic skeleton supports a healthy, dynamic, robust, responsive immune system, which in turn supports the same in the person's emotional state and life, and vice versa.

To the degree that any body system, function, or structure is not moving or showing motility, either local within itself and its direct sphere of influence, and or motility within the functional place, space, or system of which it is a part, is demonstrating a loss and or misallocation of energy, prana vitality, and orgonomic expression of life.

We must observe anything stagnant and bring movement, vitality, and stimulation to this "stuck" part, function, or quality, and encourage a return to viability and functional integrity within the living system.

Once we understand our work philosophically, we can see many ways to apply the underlying principles in practice to achieve positive outcomes for ourselves and our clients. Each distinct emphasis, systematically applied, becomes a treatment methodology in its own right.

Because our outcomes cover the gamut from Spiritual/Psyche to Emotional/Mental to Physical/Structural, i.e., the Matrix, Somatic, and Tangible Physical bodies (TPB) in all of their manifestations, the variety of expression of the work in practice and in possibility is virtually limitless.

Take this to heart. We do not come from a position or idea that we are purely constrained or limited in what we do or how we do it. This applies as long as the underlying maxim of "Do No Harm" is followed.

The 51 Systems of SomaVeda® Indigenous Thai Yoga

1) The Practical expression of loving kindness:

The primary outcomes associated with the practice of ITTM are called *"ProMiiWihan Sii"* or Four Divine, Boundless, or States of mind without limitation. They are Love, Compassion, Joy, and Equanimity. As long as these four qualities are communicated, transmitted, and exemplified during a session, we say it was good and successful. For this reason, it is possible to have a Thai Yoga session with little or even no actual touching!

In addition to the four divine states of mind we practice and perform Puja (prayer/ ritual healing) which is a multi step protocol to first Acknowledge the sacred space shared by client and healer, to honor and acknowledge the *"Boddhisatvas"* and progenitors of our way and teaching, to "Generate the Boddichitta" or perfected mental processes of enlightened beings through Mantra recitation of "*OmNamoShivago*" or Metta Sutra mantra or similar, invoking and inviting of the essences and energies of love and healing to move within the body of ourselves and our client and listening and sacred attunements.

This prayerful and thoughtful meditation and attuning to various energies and petitioning of the sacred and symbolic metaphor of deity, ancient guides, and role models, provides the basis for all further communication and expression of thoughtful ideals. Any applications of physical pressure are intended mainly to convey the Primary intentions of *"ProMiiwihan Sii"* to balance and harmonize the *"Thaat Thang Sii"* or Four Ayurveda Elements and Tri-dosha or Three Winds, Humors, and or Energetically based Body Types. Much like the physical contact of a hug can convey care, consideration, and love, the physical pressure in Traditional Thai Yoga is highly sophisticated.

2) A system of Dancing Meditation:

A movement or motion restoration system. Beginning with observing that which is not moving or which has lost the ability to contract and expand, and then restoring the living essence and function by restoring motion. Everything that's alive moves.

Every living thing that has either lost or is losing its ability to move is dying. We say that Nuad is a form of Vipassana meditation. Vipassana and or Insight Meditation finds its origin and home in the Theraveda Buddhist traditions and practices of Thailand. However, Vipassana is currently a widespread practice in many countries, including Tibet, India, Burma, Sri Lanka, Laos, Cambodia, and Vietnam, and has spread to the West through Europe and the US.

Vipassana teaches one to be mindful of the moment, every part of every part of the moment. It's famous for incorporating the so-called "walking" meditation forms.

We divide meditation forms into two primary variations... Passive- Introspective and Active Introspective. These two forms, passive or active, can be either object-focused or not. Nuad in SomaVeda® is an Active-Introspective, Dynamic, and Object-focused meditation, with the client, your relationship to the client, and your own orientation and state of mind as the meditation's objects. It can be practiced this way without focusing on any external result. When practiced in this way, both the participant and the practitioner benefit, as is common with other forms of meditation.

3) A system of Bending the Bones:

Toning, strengthening, and organizing, aligning in such a way as to stimulate, restore, strengthen, balance, and align the electrical, magnetic, circulatory, polarity, as well as increase the durability of the skeletal structures of the entire body.

Many Thai Yoga positions (Hatha Yoga Asana) exert sufficient pressure to deform or bend osseous structures, including bones. These asana and or positions range from push and pull type of techniques, such as YaNaKa or "Push the leg", to broad heavy compressive movements and positions, such as when doing "Hands Free" and "Walking or Barefoot Thai". In the hands-free variations or applications, you literally walk or stand on the client with one or both legs. As the tissue compresses and distorts, there is more than adequate pressure to bend the bones. There is substantial research suggesting that direct pressure on bony or skeletal structures can be beneficial.

4) A system of Traction and Decompression of the Skeleton:

Focusing on the joints and connective tissues of the body, including bones, ligaments, cartilage, connective tissue, and fascia. Very quickly, the practitioner learns the principle of "The highest potential for gain or loss of energy occurs at the joints." It is a hallmark and identifying feature that all Hatha Yoga and certainly facilitated Hatha Yoga styles, such as Indigenous Traditional Thai Yoga, emphasize articulation and opening (decompression) of the joints.

There are literally thousands of techniques where one pulls or pushes to create expansion and opening in every joint. There are leverage positions and rotations that do the same. Look at how Yanaka targets the knee and ankle, and how many other similar applications and positions do the same for the hip, arm, shoulder, wrist, etc.

5) A system of Pranic healing:

Bringing harmony and equilibrium of energy balance to the Matrix Body and all of its constituents or components. We say in SomaVeda® that we bring Energy, Attention, Consciousness, Breath, and Pressure to bear on each line, point, wheel, and whole person we are working with. All of these, in one way or another, target the Pranamaya Kosha, or Pranic Body (Matrix Body).

Every application or extension of energy or pressure is visualized as an extension of the breath, or one's own Prana, affecting the breath or Prana of the client. Pressure of any kind is seen as a tool for creating this focus, not as the result sought. Physical pressure can be seen from this point of view as incidental contact intentionally used to gather attention and focus the breath. This is why we say it is possible to do a session and to be effective without actually touching the client. There are many stories of our masters working entirely in this way. We say that sick or distressed areas of the body have poor or weak Prana circulation. By restoring the vital pranic body to its vibrant capacity, we see a reduction in weak or sick areas.

6) A system of Preparing For Meditation:

SomaVeda® helps support and prepare the body/ mind for the rigors and discipline of meditation and Samadhi practice. Going back to the historic Buddha himself and his Doctor and venerated student Jivaka. The Buddha ordered that this medicine be available to all monks and would have monks assist them in their study and practice. Traditionally, this work has been associated with the Theraveda Buddhist practices of Thailand (Myanmar/Sri Lanka). The idea of the practice-and-preparation religious therapeutic model is found throughout Asia and Southeast

A s i a , from Tibet to India to Burma and Thailand.

For example, we say that everyone can meditate or at least learn how to meditate. But what if you have headaches or low back pain? What if you have knee injuries or pain that hurts and distracts you if and when you try to sit still? What if you have persistent negative emotions, fears, and such that interfere with your ability to learn, etc.? What if you have no conception of how to stop moving or hold your breath, etc.?

By balancing the Dosha and Matrix body, reducing the effects of trauma and stress in the person, and reducing their overt feelings of pain and discomfort, we enable them to be more comfortable in their own skin. Now their ability to be still, to sit, to walk, and to focus for extended periods without pain allows and supports the learning and practice of meditation. Sadly, many people quit their meditation practice because they have what they feel is too much pain and discomfort. These individuals would be much more successful if they tried meditation practice after a balancing program.

7) A system of Treating Armored Points:

SomaVeda® Thai Yoga reduces the effects of armoring and armored points, and the distortion of both the Matrix and TPB that they represent. Thai Yoga accomplishes this by discerning, revealing, and treating the armoring and bio-neuro-locational aspects of negative emotions, and correcting disruptions to the body's energy system of which they are symptomatic.

Armored points have various names or different designations depending on how you look at them. They are sometimes referred to as *Lom, Marma, Muladra, Bhindi*, Trigger Points, Acupoints, Areas of High Neurologic Activity, Chakra Points, Sore Spots, Knots, Granthi, etc. We think of them as either Active or Latent. Active armored points are currently active and causing pain, discomfort, distortion, dysfunction, or all of the above in any combination, which can be seen or felt.

Latent armored points, unlike active armored points, are essentially hidden. They are causing distortion; however, it is below a conscious threshold or level of activity that is readily observable. They may be invisible to both the person who has them and the person trying to help them. Generally, though, both types of armored points are discernible if not directly, then indirectly. "By their fruits you shall know them."

To treat them effectively, they must first be observed, identified, and quantified through assessment. The primary assessment tools for locating armored points and their patterns of distortion are palpation evaluation, postural analysis (Asana), and applied kinesiology (Muscle testing/Medical Radionics).

Reducing and/or eliminating the armored points simultaneously addresses the underlying negative emotional causes, structural distortions, and disruptions and imbalances in the body's energy systems.

8) A system of Ayurveda:

Ayurveda, literally "The Art of Being" and/or "Science of Life," originating in India and Tibet, offers health maintenance and therapy, combining self-healing meditation with natural medical practice and science to facilitate healing in others. All of the Indian and Thai classic Yoga forms or systems are represented in some form or fashion, including but not limited to: Jnana, Raja, Hatha, Bhakti, Kriya, Tantra, etc. All common Ayurveda practices such as "*Marma Chikitsa, Pancha Karma, Abhyanga, Shirodara, Rasya, Sneehana*", etc. Classical Indian/Indigenous Traditional Thai Medicine (ITTM) and pharmacology, herbology, and lifestyle management are included.

Thai Ayurveda is as genuine an expression of classical indigenous Ayurveda as any other form practiced in India. Thailand was not conquered by the British or any other colonial power. For over 50 years, India suffered the depreciation and denigration, and in many cases the destruction and loss of traditional Ayurveda literature due to the strict rule of the "English" secular medicine system enforced at gunpoint. India is only now making great strides in recovering the essence of what was lost during the "Raj" period. As a Western colonial power that never conquered Thailand, it survived relatively intact. Thai Ayurveda is Ayurveda Thai Style!

For a more in-depth discussion of the history and origins of Thai Ayurveda, see the book by this author: Ayurveda of Thailand: Indigenous Traditional Thai Medicine and Yoga Therapy, Meta Journal Press, 2016; ISBN 13: 978-1-886338-05-0; available on Amazon.

9) A system of Traditional Healing with Religious & Spiritual origins:

A Religious Therapeutic system, originally based on Hindu, Buddhist, Muslim, Taoist, and Sufi traditions and teachings of making merit and reducing harmful Karma for the giver as a spiritual practice.

The definition of Karma used here is that it is the result of current and past negative, harmful, mean, or unthoughtful thoughts, actions, and deeds, as well as mechanical or formative ones. In other words, any thought, action, or deed whose origin is NOT found in the expression of *"Promiiwihan Sii"* generates harmful Karma.

One can consciously and intentionally set aims and make efforts to reduce the literal weight of so-called "Bad" Karma and obtain liberation or freedom from the cause and effect it generates in life. The actual practice of ITTM is considered a path towards liberation from bad Karma and the correction to proper alignment with God and Spirit.

The first one begins by recognizing the prison that unfettered karma creates, and the cycle of suffering it represents in one's life. Then one sets out to change it. Then one acquires practical knowledge and wisdom useful towards the aim of liberation. One then makes positive affirmations to practice discipline and awareness, the result of which is no longer participating in the origination cycle that creates suffering for oneself and others. Then this ideal model is practiced diligently in real-life circumstances to gain validation and experience.

SomaVeda® additionally incorporates the healing practices, rituals, and sacred duties of medicine persons in the Native American Indigenous Church (NAIC). Systems like SomaVeda® are dedicated attempts to organize and discipline persons to do this kind of work on themselves and to make merit by reducing the suffering of everyone else with whom we share this life and world.

10) A system of facilitated Hatha Yoga:

Both the practitioner and the client are guided to perform complementary Yoga Asanas, with the therapist as the guide and facilitator. Thai Asana is essentially similar to those found in many classical Indian Hatha Yoga systems and their literature. The Asana, or healing, postures are organized into Vinyasa or traditional Asana Flows and performed in specific sequences depending on the desired emphasis. We use a catalog of traditional Vinyasa poses, each specified for specific conditions and imbalances. Over 1000 different therapeutic postures are in the standard catalog. In practice, there is a Yin-Yang aspect to the way energy is exchanged between the client and the therapist-facilitator.

The Asanas themselves, with conscious effort, do the work of balancing the energy and posture and are equally beneficial to the facilitator as to the client. The sharing may or may not be passive and or accompanied by active resistance and/or co-facilitation. Many unique and peculiar therapeutic asanas in Thai Yoga are not commonly found in other Yoga systems. This is due in part to the special emphasis the Buddhist Sangha and temple schools placed on compassionate practice. Additionally, over the centuries, the emphasis on facilitation by one or more active partners created special attitudes and positioning that were literally impossible for even an accomplished Yogi to perform solo.

11) A system of Vipassana and or Insight Meditation:

Vipassana or Insight meditation has been taught for thousands of years by Buddhist monks from Tibet to Thailand. The emphasis is on exploring the self in pursuit of the true self. It may be practiced as a form of moving meditation as described in the Buddha Dharma, Vedic literature, and Yoga Vedanta.

Commonly illustrated as a form of "Walking or Dancing Meditation". The primary focus is to experience the insight space of Mushin, or "No Mind," while cultivating the Samadhi and Nibana/Nirvana states.

12) A system of Jnana Yoga:

SomaVeda® systematically presents and teaches the meaning, purpose, and function of life and living. By way of this teaching, the inner being of the normal, untrained, and undisciplined mind becomes honed and focused towards productive thinking, understanding, and being. Cultivation of Enlightenment and Samadhi experience is believed to be practically attainable through this practice.

13) A system of Bhakti or Devotional Yoga:

Thai Yoga is based on the concepts of Puja (prayers), Wai Khruu (paying respect), acknowledging three teachers, and acknowledging the lineage. Devotional practices may include recitation of various mantras, prostrations, burning of sacred incense, observance of altars and sacred images, and use of statuary. Devotional practices also include paying respect to living teachers, Khruu and Ajahn, who pass blessings and Shakti on to devotees. Use of healing amulets and talismans, as well as sacred objects, and the use of herbs and oils in ritual.

Traditionally, respect and devotion have been paid to the famous healer, doctor, and teacher Shivago, also known in Ayurvedic literature as Jivaka Khumarbacca. This is done in various ways, but the most common practice is reciting the Om Namo Shivago Mantra.

14) A system of teaching touch as communication:

Thai Yoga teaches touch and the art of touching with elegance and sophistication, emphasizing Non-Verbal expression of the living essence and being of one individual to another. This communication also occurs within the community, as multiple partners interact and exchange energy simultaneously. In SomaVeda®, we learn that sometimes we can communicate or express emotion and understanding more clearly through nonverbal communication and touch than through other means.

15) A system of Dynamic Facilitated Range of Motion:

All Yogic systems based on Hatha Yoga share this ability. Thai Yoga restores the vitality and function of soft tissues, fascia, and connective tissue. Reducing inner resistance to the body's own motion and increasing the range of motion. Reducing or eliminating soft tissue impingement and restriction to the healthy function of other body tissues and structures. Reducing trauma and preventing injury, etc.

16) A system of Meridian Attenuation:

Thai Yoga affects both the primary Meridians and the Trans-subcutaneous Muscle Channels (TSM), Belt Channels (Dai Mo), Connecting Vessels (Jing and Luo), and all minor connecting vessels. All primary meridians are directly addressed through postural alignments (Asana) and the use of direct and indirect pressure to acupuncture points and the meridians themselves. Meridians ad- dressed: Lung (Fei Ching), Large Intestine (Ch'ang Ching), Stomach (Wei Ching), Spleen (P'i Ching), Heart (Hsin Ching), Small Intestine (Hsiiao Ch'ang Ching), Bladder (P'ang Kuang Ching), Kidneys (Shen Ching), Heart Constrictor/ Pericardium (Hsin, Pao Le Ching), Triple Warmer (San Chao Ching), Gall Bladder (Tan ching), Liver (Kan Ching), Governing Vessel (Du Mei), Conception Vessel (Jen Mei).

17) A system of restoring consciousness to the body:

There is a concept called *"Kwan",* or the intelligence of the spirit or prana, localized to Lom/ Marma or specific points on the Tangible Physical Body (TPB). Traditionally, one cause of chronic illness affecting a specific Marma or region or specific areas or parts of the body is that, due to trauma of either mental, physical, or spiritual nature, the "Kwan" or spirit/ intelligence of that Marma or region of the body was either weakened, dislocated/ hidden, or absent.

The strengthening or restoration of Kwan, or consciousness, was achieved through Thai Yoga, thereby enhancing mind-body-emotion integration. This enhancement is facilitated by bringing Energy, Attention, Consciousness, Breath, and Pressure to Asana, Sen, Chakra, Lom, and Marma (Therapeutic Posture, Thai Sen Lines or Prana Nadi,

Chakra or wheels of light in the Matrix body, Secondary Chakra or Wind Gates, and Specific energy points, etc.). It is said we are calling the spirit (Kwan) home, as it is about bringing the spirit home and restoring vitality to what was lost or out of touch with the rest of the person.

18) A system of PranaYama (Focused Breath) Facilitation:

Every Asana focuses, guides, directs, holds, brings the breath and awareness of the breath to specific centers, organs, chakras, marma, Lom, Prana Nadi, Thai Sen Line, acupoints, and meridians. Various PranaYama techniques are used: metered breath (1, 2, 4, 7 count, etc.), mother's breath, Lion's breath, cleansing breath, releasing breath, tandem breath, etc. Visualization techniques for seeing, following, and directing the breath are also used. PranaYama can be practiced as an end in itself, as a form of personal meditation, and a path that supports the process of liberation and self-realization.

19) A system of Constructive Listening:

An organized practice of truly seeing another person as they really are. By listening, we mean a way to train and practice using every conceivable faculty to bring awareness and consciousness to bear on that which is before us. To make a connection that transcends the normal external-based experience with the very vitality and energy of another. To Hear them, to See them, to Feel them, to Breathe them, to Smell them... I use capitals to show that I mean this in a capital way, not just in the usual meaning or way that we are accustomed to. Not as untrained and unaware machines simply responding to things in a mindless, reactionary way.

When I am listening in this way, it is not as something separate and apart from the object or person of my introspection. I am more like them, and they are more like me. I start to experience the client as an extension of my own in-the-moment experience of life, and they have the same experience of me. I feel similar expressions in my own body to what they feel. My own emotional resonance and mental imagery become reflective of theirs, and vice versa.

In this way, there is an increasingly deep experience of connectedness and an inner appreciation of the limitless possibilities that life offers in its expression in every moment. I don't just hear or feel the breath; it becomes the base for an expansion of awareness, and I may be lost within its complexity. Are they breathing? Yes or no? Where is the breath? High, middle, or low? Where is the breath going? High falling, Low rising, mid space, static, or spreading? Is the breath fast or slow? Is the breath regular or irregular? Is the breath stronger on one side of the body or the other? Is there apparent symmetry?

As I listen to the breath, as an example, I see changes beginning in my own breathing. I may notice syncopation between my regular rhythms and my client's. I notice I am less apart from them. I am more connected.

20) A system of Conditioning the Nerves:

Nerve tissue in Ayurveda is described as *"Manovaha Nadi"* or Lom. Thai Yoga tones and conditions nerves and connective tissue by stimulating and stretching them, increasing proprioception and intratissue communication and function. Nerve function is also enhanced by reduced sympatheticotonia and increased oxygen and nutrient delivery to the nerves themselves.

21) A system of Organization of Healing Ideas:

Indigenous Thai Yoga, as practiced in the SomaVeda® Integrated Traditional Therapies® system knowledge base, consists of organizing principles and methodologies, psychological, spiritual, physical, and medical, belonging to specific ancient schools such as Wat Buddhai Sawan, Wat Chetuphon, Wat Mahatat, Wat Raja-Orasaram, as well as traditional Thai Medical schools such as Ayurved Vidyali and Anantasuk, Buntautuk, Sawankhalok, etc.

They include linear oral traditions passed from Master to Student for many generations over thousands of years, dating back to antiquity.

22) A system of Tao de Shen! The way of life.

The system is an alternative paradigm of life, health, and living which is holistic and based on life-affirming principles: It is an organic way of life emphasizing growth and balance, dynamic living equilibrium, and integration in harmony with all other life as opposed to the dominant Western culture's reductionist, mechanistic, self-centered, nihilistic, mechanical, brutal, and non-holistic model of the world.

The SomaVeda® way is nonviolent, communicative, green, holistic, community-minded, democratic, natural, life-affirming, loving, and sustainable. This compassionate way of life is considered the best in the world for attaining what the Buddha and other enlightened men and women described as the true medicine of the world.

23) A system of Balancing Excess and Deficiency:

It states that toxicity and or deficiency are primary causes of ill health and imbalance. It seeks to reduce toxicity and remedy deficiency. These toxicities and deficits may be any visible excess or insufficiency from energy to anxiety, to physical poisons stored in the tissue from either internal or external origin. That means symptoms may present as emotional, mental, physical, or in any combination thereof, and may be quite complex.

Generally the symptoms of ill health and imbalance, regardless of cause, look like constriction, inhibition, stagnation, excess, deficiency, rigidity, im- mobility, fixed and unresponsive or unusually sluggish, exaggerated, fractured, disintegrated, broken, arrhythmic, inappropriately sensitive, resistant, tight, spas- tic, toxic, inflamed, painful, numb and or ticklish, latent and or actively referring Trigger Points, referred and or no-local pain and sensations, low energy, tired- ness, malaise, weakness, fears, phobias and all so called psychological illness patterns and syndromes.

24) A system of Non-local or Distant Healing:

The Puja process and its application are similar to Reiki, as little or no pressure is actually necessary. Some sessions might consist entirely of Puja and affirmations. It has been demonstrated that there are treatments where the healer and/or the recipient don't need to be in the same room, city, or country, for that matter. This is akin to the "healing with Prayer" found in many Western religious traditions. Non-local treatments or sessions may be conducted using visualization and affirmation rather than contact and pressure.

Some practitioners choose to use prayer to facilitate the healing. To use SomaVeda® in this way, we try to see the client in our mind's eye and then visualize them receiving the work. Since we also believe there is merit in affirming and "agreeing" with another person's healing as a way of creating or supporting that healing process, the use of present, positive, imperative statements and affirmations is encouraged. A simple example of this might be visualizing the client and/or the client's primary issue, and making the statement, "May you be well." We are modeling the healing algorithm as presented in the Buddhist "Metta Sutra".

25) A system of Herbal Medicine and Healing:

In Thai, it is traditionally referred to as "*Nuad Prakhop Samun Prai,*" meaning "the ancient Thai way of healing with plants and herbs." Thai Yoga has an exhaustive herbal pharmacopeia comparable to that of

Traditional Indigenous Indian Ayurveda. Included in use are fresh, dried, and prepared medicines and concoctions of great variety. Additionally included are essential oils and poultices, a steamed herbal compress "Luk Prakhop," and herbs used in steams and baths.

Plants are used in both external and internal applications. In common practice, we incorporate herbs and essential oils recommended by Classical Indian Ayurveda, Thai Ayurveda, Tibetan Medicine, Native American, and Western Naturopathic Medicine. This encourages and enables the use of locally available herbs and natural medicinal substances, as well as a more eclectic and comprehensive planetary-type herbology practice.

26) A system of Medical Orthopedic, Osteopathic Physical Therapy:

SomaVeda® is excellent for the treatment and rehabilitation of injuries to bone and soft tissue. This is quite common in Thailand, and there is growing interest in the US and among Western Orthopedic Doctors, Physical Therapists, Occupational Therapists, Chiropractors, etc. Traditionally in Thailand, there was always an emphasis on healing bone and skeletal injuries, and this was practiced as a specialty called Bone Setting. Today, the average Thai Yoga practitioner focuses more on the energetic and/or soft-tissue aspects of hands-on work than on adjusting and aligning the bones, etc. In the US, most states actually prohibit non-medical persons from adjusting or correcting specific osseous subluxation of the spinal vertebrae, for example.

27) A system of Athletic and Performance Enhancement:

SomaVeda® improves flexibility, coordination, and skill, and reduces the potential for injury. It benefits pre- and post-event preparation and conditioning, as well as helps with the rehabilitation of pre-existing injuries and conditions that might reduce or interfere with performance. It is a perfect complement to all types of training regimens, including but not limited to cardiovascular, Isotonic, Isometric, weight, and strength training, martial arts, and yoga. It has been a successful part of conditioning programs as diverse as Yoga, Ballet, Pro Football, Running Sports, Tennis, Baseball, hyper-endurance sports (like Ironman), Auto Sports, Karate, Kickboxing, and Golf. SomaVeda® improves both skill and strength, and the basis of coordination and proprioception through enhanced range of motion, improved circulation, reduced adverse muscle tonicity, improved oxygen uptake in ischemic areas of poor circulation, as evidenced by oxygen deficiency, improved muscle tone, and reduction of scar tissue contracture from previous injury.

SomaVeda® enhances mind-body integration and overall ease and comfort, as well as improving post-event recovery by expediting the elimination of key wastes such as lactic acid, uric acid, tissue salts, and metabolic waste products normally generated during exercise. It increases oxygen and nutrient delivery to soft tissue, including muscle, fascia, and connective tissue. It reduces inflammation in soft tissues and edema around the joints, and also reduces sensitivity and improves the overall luster and vitality of the body. The deep relaxation aspect improves quality of life and speeds recovery, enhancing overall mental agility and durability. It may also address some performance-impacting emotional patterns.

28) A system Expressing Traditional Native Culture:

This is the colloquial and unique regional and cultural heritage and information derived from Indigenous Traditional Thai cultures, i.e., Northern (Lanna), Southern (Bangkok/ Ayudthaya), Royal (Chakri Dynasty), Hill Tribe (Karen, Akha, Lisu, Lahu, Mien, Hmaung, Pedong, Mon, etc.), as well as border-specific regional influences of the Burmese, Lao, Campochian, Malaysian, Chinese, Indian, Japanese, etc.

Each regional and/or local style acts as a repository and catalog of the unique cultural identity and heritage of that particular subgroup and its relationship to the dominant Thai Culture. The "Way of practice" is the basis of an oral tradition, teaching, or communication of core understandings, stories, metaphors, and healing methods and methodologies to each subsequent generation. A systematic passing on of values and concepts that identify and make the family, group, tribe, and region unique and special from one another. This oral tradition of passing on knowledge has been carried out over many generations, possibly for thousands of years.

We are against any procedures for "Standardization" that interfere with the unique and peculiar traditions of specific indigenous groups or peoples, tribes, and villages, etc. This common diversity of cultural expression is a vital part of the totality of Thai heritage. In other words, it's part of what makes Thai, Thai!

29) A system of Somatic education and Somatic Re-education:

SomaVeda® models, teaches, and supports balanced structure and posture, generating positive emotion and equilibrium in the body-mind continuum. It is possible to discern imbalance and illness in all parts of a person from observation of their posture alone. You can see dramatic examples of internal physical distortion and weakness, as well as emotional symptoms.

We model our emotions in our posture. Deviations from balanced postural attitudes that communicate health and vitality can often be seen even by an unpracticed eye from across the room, much less so by the trained observer. We model healthy, natural posture through facilitated asana in the client's body. This healthy modeling literally rewrites the nervous system at its most fundamental level as a training effect. Often, the greatest impediment for a client in seeing or changing their unhealthy posture is simply that. They cannot see themselves clearly or feel what the sum of their postural distortion is causing. By guiding and facilitating the client through positive and sound postural Mechanics: they have direct personal experience and, in time, can carry out the corrections on their own.

30) A system of Manual Lymphatic Drainage:

Manual Lymph Drainage techniques address edema and the inflammatory process in both chronic and acute pathological conditions resulting from either systemic or traumatic origins. SomaVeda® incorporates techniques of Complex Decongestive Therapy such as: broad deep compression, palming, joint opening and release, rolling, rocking, shaking, vibration, inversion and full body com- pression in various traditional asana, coupled with adjunct modalities of topical application of herbs, essential oils, fomentation, Pancha Karma detox regimen, therapeutic steams both conventional and Far-Infrared therapy as well as MF TDP lamps and other noninvasive tools for wellness.

31) A system of Birthing Support and Assistance:

Facilitating and assisting in the management of a healthy birth environment for both mother and baby. Includes prenatal, delivery, and postpartum techniques and applications, as well as physical, mental, and emotional support. It includes treatment forms for common conditions and pain syndromes commonly encountered by mothers. It also incorporates traditional virility treatment for fertility and sexual dysfunction for women and their partners.

32) A system of Neuromuscular Therapeutic Treatment for Pain and Suffering:

Treatment is primarily focused on syndromes characterized by active and/or latent trigger points, as well as non-local pain and pathological sensation patterns, as described by the late Dr. Janet Travell and other researchers such as Dr. Leon Chaitow and Judith Walker Delaney.

It's no accident or coincidence that many of the common locations of "trigger points", if not all of them, described as originating sources of pain and referred pain (non-local or distant), coincide with traditionally described Lom, Marma, and Acupoints.

When treated or stimulated during various Thai Vinyasa forms, the points respond positively. It appears the referral points, their corresponding pain areas (Referral zones), and any indicated related pathology do not care about the method used to deliver energy to them.

Thai traditional Vinyasa and methodology contain explicit point protocols to address pathological reflex points in every area of the body with direct and positive access.

Because of the emphasis on Asana or posture and the many virtually unlimited angles of approach, pressure can be directed on points and zones of active points with great ease and specificity, which conventional Western approaches do not support.

Thai Yoga can reasonably be expected to be effective in treating any possible variation of soft tissue pain syndrome or condition, based on the action of identifiable trigger points. (See "Trigger Points" Manual by Dr. Janet Travell, and similar source material from Dr. Leon Chaitow).

By increasing circulation of blood and oxygen to various regions of the body, reducing ischemia (low oxygen), the source of first spasm and concomitant trigger points (insertion Points of motor nerves) which cannot be directly palpated, defined explicitly, or treated effectively with peripheral point stimulation techniques, is positively affected. In other words, by using broad, non-specific, basic movements, compression, rocking, inversion, etc., to increase circulation, which brings more oxygen to whole regions of the body, oxygen deficit is reduced, and trigger points and locales of spasm are reduced or eliminated, which can be affected positively in no other way!

Broad deep pressure and compression carried through a range of motion, coupled with reduction of antagonistic muscle tension, relaxes and reduces our body's internal resistance to our own circulation and metabolic processes.

33) A system of Health Maintenance, Cancer Prevention, and Palliative Care:

The Cancer reduction and prevention model of SomaVeda® Thai Yoga is specifically related to the incidence and types of cancer that have a high or higher occurrence exclusively in chronically inflamed and or edematous tissue. Especially of interest is the application in preventing and reducing Breast Cancer in women. Specifically, Breast Care Vinyasa and therapy, or the inclusion of the breast in treatment, has always been part of Thai and other oriental based healing regimens. Also effective in addressing the possible issue of Gynecomastia or Breast Cancer in Men.

With respect to all forms of cancer, SomaVeda® emphasizes education about the importance of a plant-based diet and healthy nutrition, focusing on eating the most nutritious, organic, and locally produced foods possible. This means reducing and/or eliminating all pesticides, chemicals, and man-made, biologically manipulated "Franken Foods" from the diet. First, the practitioner is charged with becoming knowledgeable for themselves, and then with counseling and coaching their chronic disease clients to model healthier food and eating habits to achieve both resistance and longevity. We do not prescribe diets for any particular disease or medical condition. We recommend education and resources to support clients in making more appropriate and informed decisions about their own health and welfare.

Consider Indigenous, Traditional Medicinal Therapies as Cancer Complication Remediation and Palliative Support for Cachexia. Cancer and wasting (cachestic) illnesses were known to native peoples (j, k). Many different tribes and indigenous groups developed both formal and familial remedies and effective treatment strategies. Most, if not all, remedies were and are today multi-model or multi-modal in design, and implementation included emotional, spiritual, physical, and herbal, medicinal approaches. The origins of specific therapeutic approaches vary widely from one tribe to another, depending on geographic location. However, there are therapeutic approaches that meet modern criteria for effectiveness as palliative and remedial therapies.

Indigenous, traditional, and or Traditional Thai Ayurveda medicinal protocols stress a balanced lifestyle free of toxicity, with clean water (hydration), air, sunlight, natural and balanced diet (fresh, unadulterated, non-GMO foods rich in essential nutrients, EFAs, minerals), addressing psychological and emotional needs, and physical fitness. Additional benefits of indigenous Traditional Thai Medicine include non-standard, non-medical treatments for pain, inflammation, and infection. Herbs such as "*Haem*" (Thai), also known as "Tree Turmeric," among others, have been used for centuries to treat cancer, tumors, and concomitant symptoms.

Traditional/ Classical Thai Yoga/ Thai Massage contains the following areas of emphasis and therapeutic modalities, such as:

A) Sophisticated and refined Manual/ Physio/ Body-centric Hands-on interventions. It incorporates elements of energetic (unseen energy: magnetic, electric, sonic etc.) and prana assessment, mindfulness, gentle rocking, asana (positional/ postural), structural release, deep stretching, focused deep breathing or pranayama, chakra balancing (Pyscho-emotional, Somatic and proprioceptive emphasis), Prana Nadi or Sen line balancing (Lines of stress, trans-subcutaneous muscle channels, fascia and connective tissue planes and or lymphatic pathways) and rhythmic compression with either broad, deep or nonspecific tools such as palm, foot, elbow and knee to emphasize with either specific point (area of high neurologic potential) or broad trans-subcutaneous muscular or fascial plane to create a singular healing experience.

Osteo- and/or Skeletal emphasis, including "Bending the bones," stimulates the production of osteoblasts, as stress on the bones stimulates bone densification and the production of marrow factors such as stem cells and lymphocytes. Application acts as a sophisticated complex decongestive therapy, as manual lymph drainage reduces both stagnant lymph and stagnant interstitial circulation. It is both stimulating to key beneficial biochemical processes and deeply relaxing and nurturing.

Thai Yoga is a passive, assisted, and or co-facilitated, slow or non-ballistic therapy. It is non-invasive and appropriate for patients across all levels of care, including palliative, hospice, and end-of-life strategies, as well as non-medical pain management. Over 1,000 distinctive techniques have been refined and put to common use over centuries of practice.

Thai Yoga also emphasizes developing a mild, personal Yoga posture routine (personal exercise) for maintaining well-being. This type of low-impact, non- ballistic exercise meets all criteria for physical training. It is especially safe for patients, as it is self-paced and, once learned, can be practiced without supervision.

B) Nutritional and or Dietary strategies based on Classical Indo Tibetan- Burmese Ayurveda (Thai Ayurveda) and local or indigenous nutrition emphasize whole, fresh foods, unadulterated (No Chemical, processed, GMO), varietal, seasonal, and local. Nutritional emphasis includes hydration therapy, eating and meal planning, natural supplementation with herbs, minerals, salts, oils, and fats. Foods, herbs, and traditional medicines recommended or commonly used emphasize anti-inflammatory, anti-tumetic, and alkaline or anti-acid qualities. These include not only varietal and wholesome fresh vegetables but also nuts, seeds, herbs, and fresh fish high in essential nutrients, including trace minerals and EFAs.

C) Psychological/Mental and Emotional support with a nurturing counseling model. Strategies include addressing old, unresolved negative emotional issues (NEMOs/Karma) through practical, positive initiatives and activities (Metta or making Merit). Counseling strategies range from the use of prayers and singing to the recitation of positive and affirming statements, with meditation (Neuro/emotional and/or neuro-physical integration strategies). Although in traditional terms, it would be called by different names.

D) Spiritual Counseling: Origins date back to the eleventh century and earlier in Hindu and, especially, Buddhist teachings, emphasizing individual responsibility and the individual's ability to control their thoughts and inner life. Specific approaches vary according to specific individual beliefs and needs. However, the cultivation of self-awareness, self-realization, mindfulness, and the Four Divine qualities (Four boundless/ unlimited states of mind) expressed as Promiiwihan Sii (Thai Lang.) of Love, Compassion, Joy, and Equanimity (Balanced Mind) are considered paramount to the healing process of any debilitating or chronic disease, including all Cancers. Emphasis on the cultivation of high-functioning interpersonal and functional relationship dynamics, inter-family and inter-community, leads to an enhanced sense of self-worth and a reduction in Depressive symptoms. In Cancer therapy, an exemplary indication of progress is the resolution or decrease of depression/ anorexia.

34) A system of Psycho-Spiritual Mental Health:

A system of psychological, emotional, and mental restoration and balancing, emphasizing reduction of Sympatheticotonia (Wilhelm Reich) and balancing metabolic activity. SomaVeda® sees the expression of negative emotion, fears, phobias, anxiety, neurosis, psychosis, etc., as caused by or a symptom of disturbances in the body's energy system or Matrix Body. The varietal expression and manifestation of negative emotions are the effect or the result of the accumulation of past harmful karma, unresolved trauma, and sexual repression, patterns of which often begin in childhood.

These fears, phobias, anxiety, etc., are the emotional presentation of toxicity and/or deficiency (Karma), the symptom voice and/or expression of armored or blocked chakra points, Thai Lom, marma points, and trapped, blocked, stagnant, excessive, or deficient prana or chi. Additional mental and emotional disturbances can be described as a disequilibrium of Promiiwihansii (the Balance of four divine states of mind: Love, Compassion, Joy, and Equanimity).

We see all these as treatable, correctable, and manageable with the conscious, methodical application of the psychic, energetic, yogic, and meditative tools found in SomaVeda® Thai Yoga.

35) A system of Dosha Balancing:

In traditional Classical Indian Ayurveda, all people are described as exhibiting the influences of five elements: Ether, Air, Fire, Water, and Earth.

These five elemental constituents, which actually make up everything that there is, also make up the constituents of our Matrix and Tangible Physical body. However, the balance of these five elements varies for each person and follows predictable patterns at different stages of life. The three Dosha or Tri-Dosha are Vata, Pitta, and Kapha. Vata is the combination of the elements Ether and Air. Pitta is the combination of the elements and influences of Fire and Water. Kapha is the combination of the elements and influences of Water and Earth.

All of the Doshas are present all of the time. Just like all of the elements from which they are derived are present all of the time. However, not always the same and not always in the same balance or proportion of influence.

In SomaVeda® Thai Yoga, we use traditional and other methods of assessment, from palpation and pulse-taking to attitudes and general disposition, to determine the activity and balance of the Tri-Dosha, and then apply corrective balancing techniques to harmonize them more optimally, or to balance them, as is commonly said.

36) A system of Self-Healing:

SomaVeda® Thai Yoga protocols, when properly done, are as good for the giver as for the recipient. There are many positive effects of practicing for the giver. In fact, there are so many that one might be selfish and practice this healing work for self-improvement alone. Practice can be a creative way to observe oneself and bring awareness to the many different aspects of oneself. Now the client becomes a mirror with the primary focus on how the giver is while working. What do you feel? What do you think or understand? What realizations and awarenesses are present that are in normal circumstances of life not easily grasped?

Doing SomaVeda® generates a positive sense of well-being, good posture, better structure and alignment, increased energy and facilitation of breath and Prana, a compassionate expression and experience of shared of Metta (loving kindness), increased range of motion, increased circulation, meditative mind and state of being, reduced expression of negative emotions, less fear, anxiety, phobias and the like, stronger mind, healthier body and enhanced resistance to disease, connection, communication and integration with one's self and one's community. Self-practice of Hatha Yoga, including Reishi Dotton (Reishi Yoga) and Reishi Hand Yoga, provides the balance, strength, and flexibility that the TPB needs.

37) A system of Co-facilitated Hatha Yoga:

"Lazy Man's Yoga!" Co-facilitated Yoga, when applied in accordance with Ayurvedic principles, is termed "Yoga Therapy". A guided practice of Asana and Pranayama. Giving one the benefits of any regular Yoga practice. Over 1000 essential Asana or balancing postures are commonly practiced with clients. The Asana are performed in a natural, non-ballistic, non-invasive, passive, assisted range of motion with emphasis on the breath. The therapists have the option to facilitate postures in any of five distinct body positions: supine, side-lying, prone, seated, and standing.

38) A system of Hands-Free or "Walking" Yoga Therapy:

It is possible to do entire flows and Vinyasa without using the hands, thus reducing hand stress and overuse for the therapist-practitioner. Hands-free or walking Thai techniques reduce occupational disability among practitioners and enhance potential practice longevity. It reduces the impact of the size disparity between the practitioner and the client. It emphasizes gravity, posture, position, and leverage over force or strength. In practical terms, hands-free Thai means we use everything but our hands. Knees, elbows, forearms, shins, thighs, and the head are all useful tools in bringing energy, attention, consciousness, breath, and pressure to bear with the client.

Standing, kneeling, leaning, perching, walking, and sitting on the client to bring positive contact are all legitimate tools and techniques to be applied at any time.

SomaVeda® Walking Thai is characterized by applying broad, deep compression and decompression to reduce Biopathy.

All the same benefits normally ascribed to conventional, unlimited Thai are just as characteristic. One difference is that clients tend to find the stronger yet less specific application of pressure more deeply relaxing. We refer to this deep relaxation as reducing symptoms of Biopathy and/or "sympatheticotonia," and as sedating.

The Walking and "Not Hands" type of sessions' sedating effects drive clients into deep states of relaxation and Delta brain wave activity. Point work (Marma Chikitsa, Acupressure) and more specific pressure methods are generally more stimulating or tonifying.

39) A system of Therapy for the Blind and or Visually Impaired:

Thai Yoga Therapy is a traditionally chosen vocation for the visually impaired in Thailand. As so much of the work is determined kinesthetically, being blind as a practitioner implies no handicap or disability. Additionally, variations are practiced by those with various other disabilities, such as "No Hands" or "No Legs".

In SomaVeda® practice, once you have located the client, you "know" not only where the client is but also where every part of the client is! "The thigh bone is connected to the knee bone" kind of thing.

40) A system of Beauty Enhancement and Vedic Aesthetics technology:

The entire Thai vinyasa, as well as breakouts, is practiced, including reflexology of the feet, hands, neck, and shoulders; facials; detox or Pancha Karma; cleansing, purification, and scrubbing; oleation (oil massage); steam baths; use of herbs; and aromatherapy. Thai Yoga is considered at the cutting edge of health and beauty. Traditionally, Indigenous Thai Ayurveda claimed "restoring the luster and vitality and shine or healthy appearance of the complexion and body" as a significant, discernible outcome of successful treatments.

However, just because some Thai methods or techniques are excerpted from the broader repertoire does not make Thai Yoga an exclusively aesthetic and superficial practice. Nor does it take away from its energetic, spiritual, or philosophical basis.

41) A System of Correcting and Balancing PTSD:

Post-traumatic stress disorder or PTSD is an anxiety disorder characterized by persistent, frightening thoughts and memories, or flashbacks, of some ordeal or a terrifying physical or emotional event (trauma) associated with serious traumatic events and characterized by such symptoms as survivor's guilt, reliving the trauma in dreams, numbness and lack of involvement with reality, or recurrent thoughts and images. People with PTSD often feel chronically emotionally numb.

Indigenous Thai Yoga can balance the disrupted parts of the body's energy system, thereby energetically separating negative emotions and the emotional aftermath from the events that originally caused the trauma or traumatic event, so that they are stored within the person's mind, emotions, and tissues via the process of armoring. The nurturing and balancing touch brings the person home, so to speak, to the present reality of life and consciousness, substituting negative emotional patterning with healthy, positive patterning.

Although it is not unusual for clients to experience some degree of emotional or physical catharsis, it is not a normal part of treatment design. It is an artifact of the powerful emotional release clients often experience during and after a series of one or more sessions.

Considering the state of the world and the prevalence of traumatic events in life, especially for both soldiers and for survivors of violent physical and or emotional abuse, it is possible to design a practice entirely targeting these types of individuals.

42) A system of Ayurveda Pancha Karma:

Pancha Karma means Five Cleansing Actions. Pancha Karma literally means "The five cleansing actions" and refers to the removal of harmful residues from past life, both current and pre-incarnate. We also take it to mean a five-step program of detoxification and purging harmful influences from the body, such as chemical residues, poisonous waste, toxins, pollutants, and perhaps various parasitic elements as well. Additionally, the Pancha Karma treatment is invigorating and stimulating to the immune system and overall vigor and vitality for the whole person. It is relaxing, rejuvenating, nurturing, and spiritually uplifting. Although it is a SomaVeda® Thai Yoga and Classical Vedic healing practice with energetic and spiritual origins, it is perhaps also the ultimate origin of most Western "Spa" type treatments practiced today. Pancha Karma is the original hygiene system, predating even Roman and Turkish Baths by as much as 1000 to 2000 years!

There are basically five individual steps or processes common to each Thai Yoga Pancha Karma program. These are a bit simpler, condensed versions of the full-blown, lengthy, and equipment-intensive Pancha Karma we teach in India through our Ayurvedic Residential Pancha Karma Specialist Programs. The Classical Indian Pancha Karma is designed for a special clinical setting with very specific requirements and equipment. Our Thai version is quite simple and designed to be performed just about anywhere, and with minimal equipment. Most of the necessary equipment can actually be "Home Made"!

The point is to emphasize the nature of the treatment and the desired outcomes, and to create an accessible program that every client can receive.

Five Pancha Karma steps common to SomaVeda® Indigenous Thai Yoga:

A) Phaen Boran Ráksãa Thaang Nûat: (Mat work: A short general session. SomaVeda® Level One is perfect.)

B) Swedana: Steam or Sweat:

a. Steam session with Aromatherapy element. Thai Chair: Body, Scalp, and Facial, Steam session chair with Aromatherapy.

b. Steam session with Aromatherapy element. Steam session on a table or chair with Aromatherapy.

C) Kratop Session: Application/ Anointing with Sacred Herbs: Exfoliation and body wash with herbs or earth minerals, wet or dry.

D) Snehana: Oleation Session:

a. Abhyanga: Anointing with single or multiple therapists.
b. Body Wrap
c. Nasya: Sesame oil nasal therapy.

E) Shirodhara: Oil and/or Aroma Therapy Drip on the forehead.

43) A system of Healing and Nurturing Animals:

We have extensively observed and documented the positive effects of SomaVeda® Thai Yoga on animals. The author and his wife have performed very complete sessions on an ailing Greyhound puppy for over 6 years, with great benefit. We have seen practitioners work with dogs, cats, and even horses! I once rescued an injured hawk and began treating it using a Thai Yoga technique.

The first key is to emphasize the energy over Asana, as many postures might be difficult or impossible with some animals, of course! You can do Puja for and with any living thing. From there, think in practical terms. For small animals, perhaps you can gently guide them into various positions to access the lines and points. One thing to consider is that the Matrix body outline and constituents are the same for a horse or dog as they are for you!

44) A system of Brotherhood/ Sisterhood:

Question? What is a Christian equivalent to the concept of "Sangha"?

A Sangha or Men and women dedicated to practicing "*Ahimsa Dhamma*", or nonviolent acknowledgment of the sanctity of life and all living beings. This is as described in the Metta Sutra and other philosophical and sacred texts, to work for the betterment and reduction of suffering for all living beings. Thai Yoga provides a practical method for individuals working together to "No longer participate in the origin cycle of the creation of suffering" for ourselves and those around us.

Our community, through the singular expression of our feelings and beliefs and the use of concrete methodologies, provides a workable example of the Way of Right Livelihood. We share a way, a path of living and working which provides us with guidance, moral and ethical principles as well as nurturing support and comfort. Within our Sangha, we share all the divine or at least noble principles of love, compassion, joy, and equanimity.

45) A system of Differential Diagnosis and Indigenous Ayurveda Assessment:

Thai yoga may be used, in part or in full, as a systematic approach to assessing and qualifying states of health or imbalance, and as a sound template for devising strategies to correct imbalance. Actually, conducting a session provides an opportunity to perform a thorough head-to-toe assessment for the client. Virtually every area of the Spirit, Mind, and Body is closely inspected.

The following classic Thai Yoga Therapy assessments can be made:

- What Kosha or Energy Body is the primary or source of imbalance?
- Dominance of Gunas: Satvas, Rajas, and or Tamas attribute.
- Male or female indication, such as Yin or Yang inclination in imbalance.
- What Dhatu or Element or combination of elements is indicated?
- What Organ of Action, Function, or Sense is indicated?
- What Orifice is indicated? (Relation of Orifice to Sen line)
- Which Dosha, Vata, Pitta, or Kapha is indicated in imbalance (Vikruti)?
- Reading the Vedic Pulse: Vata, Pitta, or Kapha
- What Sen Line or Prana Nadi is indicated?
- What Chakra is indicated?
- What are the Asana and or postural indications?
- Assessment by Palpation evaluation
- Trigger Point and or Sensitive Point Assessment

- Inflammation and or edema assessment.
- Indication of Emotional or Armored points.
- Range of motion assessment
- Reflex assessment
- Prana and Breath Assessment
- Key Lom and or Marma Assessment
- Primary Complaint Assessment
- Type of Disruption to the body's energy system: Negative emotional patterns, i.e., phobias, compulsions, etc. (Old Unresolved Negative Emotional Issues: NEMOs, Energy Toxins)

46) A system of Expression of Religious Freedom and Free Speech:

Sharing this work provides a dynamic and ever-expanding vocabulary for expressing ideas and philosophies about what we believe is true and who we are or want to be in life. It is the practical expression of loving-kindness and love, by definition. We believe that love manifests not as some mystical, ephemeral, intangible moral concept but as a genuine, life-affirming communication of care and consideration.

By its rationale of serving both the giver and the receiver, it expresses organic, democratic, and natural values that are equally beneficial to individuals, families, communities, and the greater world.

The Puja, Wai Khruu, and Yogic Vinyasa forms provide a health-and-healing exchange of core values among all persons engaged in their practice. The world is a better place because it exists and would be less so without it. It is a sure cure, an antidote for pain and suffering, whether of Psychic, spiritual, emotional, physical, or environmental origin. Even if one were to discount all spiritual or energetic considerations entirely, it would still provide a long list of positives.

This work perfectly expresses the aspirations and admonitions not only of the historical Buddha but also of all genuine saints and sages who, out of obligation to their religious expression, have contributed to our practices. We join this contemplative community by using every faculty of mind, body, and spirit to speak, to counsel, to express our beliefs with freedom of expression.

Religious Therapeutics is just one of many ways to put the tenets of our religion into practice. The tenants that clearly say to administer, to succor, to comfort, to heal, to restore, and to cure.

47) A system of Chakra Based "Korosot" Astrology:

SomaVeda® Chakra Astrology is based on the fifty-two correlations for each of the seven primary chakras. Each Chakra has both traditional planetary and numerological associations, which are cyclical.

Basically, the theory is that each primary Chakra and planet rules or exerts an overriding influence for seven years, divided into seven smaller yearly cycles. This is discussed in detail in the book "Lines, Wheels, Points and Specific Remedies" by this same author.

Furthermore, there is a secondary system of Chakra body types and or Chakra personality types. The Chakra body types further support the differentiation of the Vedic Doshas.

See the book "Korosot Chakra Astrology". "Chakra Poster" or "Lines, Wheels, Points and Specific Remedies" for specific details for each Chakra and the method for doing a SomaVeda® Chakra Korosot Reading.

48) A System of Tantra:

Often misunderstood, Tantra is a Classical Indian/Indo-Aryan Sanskrit word literally meaning "expansion through awareness". It includes teachings and practices that use energy to lead to a high state of enlightenment and blissful existence. Ayurveda, as an Indigenous Religious Therapeutic Healing Science, also incorporates the ancient Tantric text and commentaries.

SomaVeda® Thai Yoga can be a spiritual path that uses all of the sense faculties, breath, sounds (Mantra, tones), movements (Asana), and various symbols (Chakra Yantra) to bring peace to the mind and to activate sexual energy (Kundalini Shakti), focusing and directing it throughout the mind, body and spirit of the person to to achieve specific states of consciousness and bliss.

These understandings were originally part of the ancient meditative and healing practices of India, Tibet, Nepal, Thai, and Chinese cultures. In the ancient past, they may have been reserved for the training of royalty, spiritual adepts, and sages; however, the teachings and practices are now available to everyone. The Thai style derives primarily from the Vedic and Taoist cultures.

These practices (Pranayama, Asana, Vinyasa, Visualization, etc.) coupled with sensitive, loving, and sensual touch can also help heal past trauma and emotional injuries stored in the sexual centers or Chakras of the body.

By opening the Chakra and Sen or Nadi's of the body, it is possible to be more fully available and in the moment with your expression of love and expression of your true sexual nature. Kundalini, or the vital life force of Prana, is considered the only energy we can consciously control or direct, with the potential to create or facilitate life.

By creating the possibility to cultivate, gather, direct, and share this Kundalini energy, we can bring life to every part of us. Bring vital energy to the mind, body, and spirit. Bring vital healing energy to the sick or injured parts of us.

When practiced with a willing partner, the atmosphere and connections created can bring about powerful flows of connection and energy. These empower you to expand your love for one another and for all living beings.

Thai Yoga Tantra balances the male and female energies (Yin and Yang) within your person and with and between you and your partner. The sacredness and divine practice of intentional union break down the normal barriers and inner constraints that limit the free expression of perfect union, making every touch, breath, and movement a divine gift. We honor our divine male and female energies as perfected expressions of the sacred within us.

There are practices suitable for both single (solo) cultivation and cultivation by partners and couples.

IMPORTANT NOTE: We recommend that overt sacred sexual activity of any kind only occur between informed and consenting adults and never in a professional healing setting.

49) A System of TOBIN Integrated Immunity Protocol

SomaVeda® Thai Yoga-Ayurveda and Integrative Health, TOBIN Protocol, and Tridosha.

I plan to introduce new concepts you may not have heard before and to refresh your thinking about SomaVeda® Thai Yoga-Ayurveda in a modern, creative, and fresh way. It's about bridging ancient wisdom and modern immunity. Okay, so without further ado, I'm going to jump into my presentation, which will be urgent and precise.

At a microscopic level, human biology is currently under an assault it never evolved to withstand. Synthetic, jagged microparticles are breaching organic cell membranes, the invisible fallout of our industrial age. For over

5,000 years, classical SomaVeda® Thai Yoga-Ayurveda served as a primary defense against illness.

It is a terrain-based medical system optimized for treating root causes through Tridosha theory, mapping the human body as an integrated network of energetic and metabolic pathways. But the 21st century has introduced novel synthetic vectors. Endocrine disruptors, PFAS chemicals, and genetically modified organisms present chemical signatures that did not exist during SomaVeda® Thai Yoga-Ayurveda's inception.

Modern Western allopathy attempts to manage these chronic vectors through acute crisis management, relying heavily on chemical suppression. By prescribing psychotropics or broad-spectrum antibiotics to manage symptoms, this allopathic suppression can disrupt the biological terrain further, often creating a cycle of iatrogenic harm. Western medicine focuses on the seed, the specific pathogen or symptom.

SomaVeda® Thai Yoga-Ayurveda prioritizes the soil, the overall biological terrain. To maintain clinical efficacy against modern toxins, Ayurvedic practitioners are increasingly adopting a two-eyed seeing framework by integrating Dr. Benoit Tannot's TOBIN protocol. Surviving the modern era requires anchoring ancient sensory diagnostics in modern integrative immunological data.

In SomaVeda® Thai Yoga-Ayurveda, health is rooted in Agni, the body's digestive and metabolic fire. This internal intelligence evolved over millennia to process natural organic inputs. When the biological terrain is presented with recognizable biological matter, Agni processes these inputs to extract nutrients and maintain systemic balance.

SomaVeda® Thai Yoga-Ayurveda classifies the accumulation of environmental poisons as Garavisha. Today, global industrial practices have scaled this threat to a volume that overwhelms ancestral metabolic pathways. Modern synthetic substances and heavy metals act as unintelligent inputs.

They confuse the metabolic fire, causing Agni to falter and dim. The biological consequence of this metabolic confusion is the systemic accumulation of Ama, a toxic metabolic residue that bypasses normal filtration and spreads throughout the tissues. Traditional sensory diagnostics, such as reading the pulse or analyzing the tongue, detect this accumulation.

They cannot, however, identify the specific invisible synthetic agents causing the blockage. Without identifying the specific synthetic vector, the practitioner lacks the diagnostic resolution required to clear the biological terrain at its source. Dr. Benoit Tano's TOBIN framework addresses this gap.

It is a root-cause systems biology model designed specifically for integrative immunity. TOBIN breaks down into five actionable pillars: toxicity, oxidative stress, biological and hormonal imbalance, infections and inflammation, and nutrient deficiencies. These five pillars encompass the upstream drivers of nearly all modern chronic diseases and immune dysfunction.

TOBIN functions alongside Tridosha theory and traditional assessment, providing a specific immunological layer to the existing diagnostic process. For the advanced practitioner, TOBIN serves as a functional pathology vocabulary. It allows healers to quantify and track modern disease drivers, such as microscopic forever chemicals that evade the naked eye.

This biochemical data provides a bridge, validating classical ayurvedic imbalances for Western medical peers through the lens of systems biology. We can construct a direct translation matrix to bridge Western integrative immunology and Eastern bioenergetics. The "T" for toxicity maps directly to "*AMA*" and "*Garavisha.*"

Environmental toxins trigger chronic immune responses that disrupt the body's natural baseline. This impact is seen across the doshas. Toxicity localized in Pitta causes systemic hypersensitivity and allergic reactions, while in Vata, it drives neurological distress and erratic pain.

As seen in this diagram of the pranas, the "B" for biological imbalance maps to grihani roga and disrupted apana value in the lower abdomen. This correlates with the Western concept of leaky gut syndrome, in which compromised barriers allow endotoxins to enter the bloodstream. The O for oxidative stress and the I for inflammation and infections map directly to Pitta derangement.

Resolving this specific biochemical fire is a prerequisite to rebuilding "*Ojas*", the subtle essence of long-term tissue health and immunity. Finally, the N for nutrient deficiencies maps to kapha imbalances, linking poor nutrition and endocrine disruption to profound cellular fatigue. Every immunological biomarker identified in the TOBIN protocol has a precise, actionable equivalent in classical TriDosha pathology.

In a clinical setting, a practitioner operationalizes this mapped data to move beyond generic protocols. First, they gather traditional inputs, the innate constitution, or prakruti; the current state of illness, or vikruti; the Vedic pulse; and the kosha evaluation. Simultaneously, they pull in modern diagnostic inputs, including oxidative stress panels, microbiome sequencing, and comprehensive hormone assays.

These datasets are synthesized to isolate the core deviation from the patient's baseline and identify the exact point at which the doshas have diverged. This directs the primary clinical strategy. The treatment targets this specific, quantified deviation rather than the patient's baseline constitution.

This precision avoids the allopathic trap of prescribing psychotropics to suppress anxiety, when that anxiety is actually rooted in a toxic vata and gut derangement. It also resolves the probiotic paradox found in functional medicine, attempting to seed the gut with bacteria, without correcting the biochemical terrain they require to survive. Operationalizing TOBIN provides a methodology for identifying the precise biochemical roots of a dosha imbalance.

When targeted terrain intervention is built on a combined diagnostic model, it can address the source of turbulence directly. Tridosha remains a highly effective functional pathology framework for mapping human health. The TOBIN protocol provides the high-resolution data necessary to apply Tridosha principles effectively within a modern, toxic environment.

Adopting modern immunological diagnostics reinforces traditional Ayurvedic wisdom by providing a clear view of today's unique environmental burdens. This integration fulfills SomaVeda® Thai Yoga-Ayurveda's core philosophical mandate, treating the patient's exact bio-individual reality with the most precise tools available. The clinical goal is to move patient care beyond the cycle of managing symptoms with chemicals.

Mastering two-eyed seeing restores the biological terrain, offering true root-cause resolution and returning health sovereignty to both practitioner and patient. I hope that you found the first short presentation overview on my topic, SomaVeda® Thai Yoga-Ayurveda and Integrative Health, TOBIN Protocol, and Tridosha, interesting. It's kind of a down-and-dirty, 10,000-foot overview of what I'm now going to dive into in part two, a little more deeply

The core theme of my presentation, unifying our 5,000-year-old classical Ayurvedic wisdom with the cutting-edge science of modern integrative immunology, I'm using and recommending Dr. Benoit Tano's TOBIN Protocol as a scientific bridge concept to translate ancient insights for the 21st century. I want you to consider, in contrast, the pristine world of the ancient Ayurvedic text against today's compromised environment. Our modern world, our biological terrain, is heavily burdened by novel or unique synthetic stressors.

What I mean by synthetic stressors is artificially man-made environmental toxins. PFAS, GMOs, pesticides, ultra-processed diets, iatrogenic harmful substances used in medicine, antibiotics, chemotherapy, radiation, chemicals, drugs, ELF, EMF, hard radiation isotopes such as cesium and plutonium that the ancients never encountered.

Can you imagine that Atria or the forefathers of SomaVeda® Thai Yoga-Ayurveda, the authors of the Charaka Samhita, the Sushruta Samhita, the

Harapika, etc., etc., that they would have rolled in their graves that we're in such a dystopian fantasy version of what they might imagine that the world would be at this time and in this day? We're under influences from every side they never imagined, and we have to take what they gave us as functional, practical medicine and adapt it to a contentious modern environment called the 21st-century biological terrain.

Let's start with the fundamentals. One of the fundamental reasons SomaVeda® Thai Yoga-Ayurveda is often overlooked as part of a holistic or integrative medical strategy, especially here in the U.S. or in the West, is that we have this foundation in energy. Well, the Western docs do too.

They choose not to emphasize it. Energy and matter exist on the same continuum. Human physiology is simply the physical manifestation of God's original consciousness, expressed through the five universal forces: ether, air, fire, water, and earth.

So we're literally describing what the Western medical world calls alchemy. It's not alchemy in that sense. It's a practical manifestation, practical physics, more on a quantum interpretation level, but practical and usable all at the same time.

Of course, I know that. As an Ayurvedic practitioner, you also know that strict elemental sequences are driving metabolic function, Vata, ether, and air, for movement and the nervous system.

Pitta, fire, and water, for thermal energy and digestion. And Kapha, water and earth, for potential energy and structure. And this is not random or chaotic.

In SomaVeda® Thai Yoga-Ayurveda, we speak of the clinical cascade of disease that begins with the elemental imbalance. Actually, it begins further back than that, right? The Charaka Samhita discusses the separation from the knowledge of oneness with God as the origin of disease. But then we get into the cascade, which is the manifestation of ego differentiated into five elements, beginning with the weakened metabolic fire, or "*Agnimandhya*", which causes the accumulation of toxic residue, or Ama, ultimately leading to immune collapse and tissue burnout, or Ojas depletion.

Here is the Western counterpart that aligns with what I just described: how we can unite our energy-based beliefs with Western medical, biologically based beliefs. And it's through the interpretation of metabolism and the immune system.

So, I want to introduce you to the TOBIN Protocol, T-O-B-I-N. Like SomaVeda® Thai Yoga-Ayurveda, this modern framework rejects symptom suppression in favor of restoring the terrain by addressing upstream drivers of disease.

Like SomaVeda® Thai Yoga-Ayurveda, TOBIN is a terrain-based model, a scientifically-based terrain model, not a reductionist Western medical model. "T.O.B.I.N", or TOBIN, is the acronym that describes what drives chronic disease expression. T for toxin overload, O for oxidative stress, B for biologic and hormonal imbalance, I for infections and inflammation, and N for nutrient deficiencies.

Now, I know many of you Ayurvedic professors and many of you Ayurvedic physicians know that some or all of these things are important. Still, you may struggle to find their exact expression in classic SomaVeda® Thai Yoga-Ayurveda literature, which is translated, of course, or in the way that you were maybe originally taught. I want to help simplify that. Now, we have the TOBIN framework to act as the bridge concept.

TOBIN bridges the gap of SomaVeda® Thai Yoga-Ayurveda understanding of Ama and *"Garovesha"* and the Western concept of toxicity. TOBIN's environmental toxins, heavy metals, and GMOs correlate directly with Ama and "*Garovesha*". Note the clinical manifestation in the example.

When this toxicity settles in Pitta, the Ama and *"Garovesha,"* it drives systemic hypersensitivity. In Vata, it drives neurologic stress and erratic pain. You get it? The modern Western medical diagnosis of gut dysbiosis, which by the way is epidemic, it's endemic, epidemic, it's everywhere in the world now, I think it is a side effect also of the COVID vaccine and boosters.

Leaky gut is equivalent to the disruption of "*Apanavayu*" and comprises compromised "*Grahani*", the intestinal barrier. As an example, the clinical insight, indiscriminate high-dose probiotics uselessly plant seeds in the toxic soil. We must clear the Ama first.

We must first improve the quality of the soil. And yes, I prescribe probiotics. I even make my own brand of probiotics.

But is it a panacea for gut dysbiosis, leaky gut, and Crohn's disease? And the answer is no. No, it's not. And in fact, you might think it should work.

The client starts taking probiotics, but they don't get better. And you have to understand that, according to more classical SomaVeda® Thai Yoga-Ayurveda, it's because we did not prepare the soil first. We did not clean, clear, or prepare the soil to be a good home for the probiotic seeds.

TOBIN compares chronic immune hyperactivity and cellular damage to classic Pitta derangements. The ultimate goal is to resolve these immunological fires to restore Ojas, the subtle essence of tissue health. That's the goal.

Now let's go on. TOBIN sees Kapha stagnation as the result of ultra-processed diets and endocrine disruptors creating cellular starvation, which manifests energetically as Kapha stagnation, sluggishness in the Srotas. Treat this by utilizing warming, drying therapies to reignite the fire, lightening therapies to reignite the fire.

Both Western medical and Ayurvedic understandings can define the very same observed conditions or symptoms. It's worth noting that SomaVeda® Thai Yoga-Ayurveda is stronger on the energy and less-tangible, qualitative side of analysis and assessment. In contrast, the TOBIN-style protocol is stronger on the terrain milieu or biological side. Both sides are complementary and support the overall goal of restoring health to the sick.

Now, this slide is a quick summary table. It shows how practitioners can look at a Western mechanism like ROS or leaky gut and instantly translate it to its Ayurvedic equivalent and primary Dosha impact.

Now, I want to go over five reasons I believe SomaVeda® Thai Yoga-Ayurveda practitioners should adopt the TOBIN methodology. Number one, it adds validation through systems biology.

It enhances diagnostic precision. It manages 21st-century pathologies. Remember, we're under adverse influences, what in TCM they call evil influences that never existed at the time of the ancient Rishis who first created SomaVeda® Thai Yoga-Ayurveda.

And in fact, many of them didn't exist in the world until the 1930s and the 1940s, literally post Second World War, 21st-century pathologies. Restoring the three restores the biologic terrain and the patient's health sovereignty. We want to do anything we can to give our clients better, more trustworthy sources for their own health and wellness, and for the future of their health and wellness for them and their families.

Well, that's going to make us famous, and that is our mission, right? That is our mission. TOBIN translates our traditional principles into the language of modern genomics and functional immunology, enabling us to communicate confidently with our Western medical peers. This is important.

TOBIN integrates modern specific biomarkers, i.e., what are biomarkers? They're tests. They're the lab tests that Western hospitals and clinics are so fond of overusing. But we're not Luddites; we don't believe that testing is, in and of itself, a bad thing.

We believe that random, chaotic, endless testing to generate income for a clinic, hospital, or practitioner is wrong and harmful. So we want to zero in on the biologics that can be helpful, and TOBIN can give you a blueprint on what those are and how to use them. Oxidative stress markers, for example.

With our traditional pulse and tongue assessments, which I love, we can use them alongside the biologics to pinpoint the exact biochemical manifestations of dosha imbalance. This is the important part. I can correlate a dosha imbalance with a biochemical manifestation, and I can do so in three dimensions using a scientific lab test.

It's why I have a darkfield microscope in my clinic. There are limitations to SomaVeda® Thai Yoga-Ayurveda practice today. I'm not being critical, and I don't say this as criticism.

It's just a statement. There are limitations. Classical SomaVeda® Thai Yoga-Ayurveda didn't have to deal with the air pollution, synthetic chemical industry, EMF, ELF, chemtrails, radioactive isotopes, xenoestrogen plasticizers, microplastic contaminated landscape of the modern world.

Did not have to deal with it, so they didn't know about it, and there are no classical Indian remedies in the Charaka Samhita for detoxing xenoestrogen plasticizers or Cesium-123. TOBIN provides the necessary upgrade to understand how novel toxins work, specifically target "*Agni*" and "*Ojas*" today. In both TOBIN and SomaVeda® Thai Yoga-Ayurveda, we emphasize treating and correcting the soil, not the weeds.

Preventing iatrogenic harm, as caused by standard treatments and antibiotics, requires an integrated approach to resolve the root cause. TOBIN is still all about the root cause. I want to encourage you to move past the one-size-fits-all model, if you have it.

Empower your patients with personalized, data-based treatment plans that combine ancient wisdom with lab-verified progress.

Two-Eyed Seeing

Why two-eyed seeing? Two-eyed seeing, is a Native American saying, and what it refers to is human beings, upright two-legged, human beings have two eyes, a left and a right eye.

Believe it or not, the world that the left eye sees is not the same as the world the right eye sees. Now take your hand and cover your left eye, then look at the screen for a minute, okay? Now cover your right eye, look at the screen for a minute, and realize that what you see is not the same from one side to the other, from one eye to the other. But when you open both eyes, you see something that looks solid, that looks the same, but it's different than what you saw with the left eye and what you saw with the right eye.

If SomaVeda® Thai Yoga-Ayurveda is our left eye and TOBIN is our right eye, when we take these two methodologies and apply them, looking with both eyes, we see something more comprehensive and cohesive than we could before. And also, I'm going to say it again, okay? Don't take my advocacy and recommendation of the TOBIN framework as being critical of SomaVeda® Thai Yoga-Ayurveda in any way. I define myself as an SomaVeda® Thai Yoga-Ayurveda practitioner.

Tridosha is the original functional pathology framework, and I teach Tridosha in every SomaVeda® Thai Yoga-Ayurveda program that I teach, now going on 42 years. By integrating the TOBIN protocol, we wield cutting-edge science to defeat chronic disease, reclaim the terrain, treat the soil, and restore "*Ojas*". So now we can see the bridge of integrative immunity, which provides a beautiful visual summary of how the bioenergetic drivers map to the TOBIN pillars.

49) A system of Battlefield Acupuncture-Acupressure "SVTD-BFA" Protocol

How BFA Fits into the SomaVeda® TAELR Strategy

The integration of Battlefield Acupuncture (BFA) into the SomaVeda® Tool Assisted Energy Line Release (TAELR) strategy represents a sophisticated synthesis of "top-down" central nervous system stabilization and "bottom-up" somatic release.

How BFA Fits into the SomaVeda® TAELR Strategy In the SomaVeda® framework, health is evaluated through the flow of Prana along energy lines (Sip Sen) intersecting at vital points (Marmas). The five auricular points of the BFA protocol, Cingulate Gyrus, Thalamus, Omega 2, Point Zero, and Shen Men, act as highly concentrated **"Auricular Marmas"**. Because Sen Lawusang and Sen Ulangka directly terminate at the left and right ears, utilizing non-invasive TAELR tools (like Piezo pens, electro-acupuncture, or magnetic pellets) on these points effectively "tunes" these specific energetic pathways.

When applied at the beginning or end of a SomaVeda® Thai Yoga Therapeutic Day Program (STDP), BFA serves as a **"neurological anchor."** It induces immediate autonomic homeostasis and pain reduction, which allows the client to participate much more comfortably in the physically demanding manual stretching, Asana positional releases, and rhythmic compressions of the session.

Opening Doors to Hard-to-Achieve Remedies Adding the BFA TAELR protocol to the SomaVeda® tool chest allows practitioners to achieve results that are often impossible with manual therapy alone. While Thai Yoga massage warms the body, improves joint mobility, and clears surface-level myofascial knots, BFA chemically suppresses pain at the spinal cord level and triggers the release of endogenous opioids (like beta-endorphins). This dual approach addresses deep-seated neurological pain patterns and connective tissue issues that standard physical manipulation cannot reach, resulting in a synergistic **"full-body release"**.

Impact on Extreme Pain, PTSD, and Veteran Health BFA was specifically designed by military physicians to provide rapid, highly effective pain attenuation in combat settings without the lethargy or addictive risks of opioid narcotics. For Veterans and patients dealing with severe PTSD, the integration of BFA is life-changing:

- **Fear Extinction and Trauma Release:** PTSD traps the nervous system in states of hyperarousal or dissociation. BFA modulates the brain's limbic system and has been clinically shown to significantly enhance the extinction of learned fear and reduce startle responses.
- **Autonomic Reset:** Stimulating points like Omega 2 and Shen Men activates the parasympathetic nervous system and the vagus nerve, counteracting the chronic "fight or flight" sympathetic drive. This creates an internal "island of safety," reducing procedural anxiety so trauma survivors can process physical touch and somatic release without being re-traumatized.
- **Mental Health:** Chronic pain is frequently comorbid with depression and anxiety. By promoting the release of serotonin and dopamine while suppressing pro-inflammatory cytokines, BFA directly targets the neurochemical roots of emotional distress and fatigue.

Addressing Specific Physical Conditions Because BFA interacts with the brain's primary sensory relay station (the thalamus) to gate ascending pain signals, it drastically expands the scope of conditions a SomaVeda® practitioner can successfully manage:

- **Back Pain and Trauma:** BFA demonstrates significant efficacy for acute and chronic musculoskeletal pain, including low back pain and limb trauma. Rapidly removing the sensation of pain allows patients recovering from accidents to actively engage in their physical rehabilitation.
- **Recovery from Surgery:** Clinical studies show that BFA significantly reduces postoperative pain intensity and decreases the need for post-surgical opioid consumption following procedures like shoulder surgeries and tonsillectomies.
- **Abdominal and Pelvic Pain:** Auricular therapy is widely utilized to modulate inflammatory markers and neural excitability in the treatment of chronic pelvic pain, endometriosis-related pain, and acute abdominal pain (such as biliary colic).

Ultimately, adding the non-invasive SV-TD BFA TAELR protocol provides SomaVeda® practitioners with a predictable, legally protected, and highly effective alternative to conventional drugs, offering a complete blueprint to transition patients from chronic depletion and trauma into lasting vitality.

50) A system of SomaVeda® TAELR: Tool Assisted Energy Line Release

SomaVeda® TAELR: Tool Assisted Energy Line Release is a comprehensive therapeutic system that incorporates physical instruments and devices to extend, amplify, and enhance a practitioner's ability to balance a client's energy toward homeodynamic equilibrium. These "tools" can be made of any material, may be electronic, and can utilize any natural energy—such as light, sound, water, or magnetic frequencies—provided the application is entirely non-invasive and causes no harm.

Central to the TAELR protocol is the systematic application of percussive energy to the body, which includes rhythmic tapping, slapping, knocking, or striking along the energetic pathways, such as the Thai Sen lines, Prana Nadi, meridians, Marma points, and Chakras. This percussive stimulation is designed to release toxins from tissues, restore circulatory flows, reduce localized inflammation, and even stimulate bone marrow production.

Beyond physical restoration, TAELR serves a profound spiritual function within Indigenous Traditional Thai Ayurveda. Tapping and striking are used to address chronic issues viewed as a deficiency or absence of the body's spirit or consciousness (*Kwan*) in a specific area. By stimulating these regions, practitioners perform the action of "Calling the Spirit Home" (*Tham Maat Kwan Baan*), restoring vital consciousness and intelligence to the affected part.

TAELR methodologies are highly integrative and can be seamlessly combined with Traditional Thai Nuad on a mat, table, or chair. The system embraces a global approach to healing, adopting tools from any culture as long as the core intention remains focused on energy balancing. This includes the integration of protocols like Battlefield Acupuncture (BFA), where tools like Piezo pens or magnetic pellets are used on auricular Marmas to create a "neurological anchor," effectively gating pain signals and facilitating deep somatic and trauma release.

Examples of SomaVeda® Preferred TAELR Tools:

- Comprehensive Assessment using Biological analysis (i.e., St. John POC)
- Yoga Therapy Props, Pillows, and Bolsters of various sizes
- Sound and frequency Therapy (Singing Bowls, Bells, and Tuning Forks)
- BIA, Bioimpedance Analysis
- PULSE XL PRO PEMF

- Hyperbaric Chamber (mHBOT)
- LifeTimeVibe® Whole Body Vibratory Therapy
- Chakra Bio-Mat® (Full Spectrum Crystal Mat with LF PEMF, Far Infrared, and Red Light Therapy)
- PhotoBioModulation (Red Light or Bioptron Hyperlight Spot Application)
- Colored Goggles: Colored Light Therapy
- MFTDP Mineral Lamp with Far-infrared Light
- RSMIBEA® 2400w PhotoBioModulation (Full Body Red Light)
- 4D Triton Massage Chair (Thai, Shiatsu, or Zone-Based Compression AI Protocol)
- David Pro Mind-Gym or MindTap® (Binaural Audio-Light Neuro-entrainment)
- Jade Vitatron® Iontophoretic Foot Bath (Non-invasive Detoxification and infusion)
- Russian Vitafon (Vibro-acoustic, Micro-acoustic, Audio-Vibrational Frequency Sound Therapy)
- Jade Vital Therapeutics (Electro-homeopathic Formulations)
- Beck Protocol: Ozone Water, Colloidal Silver, Micro-pulsing-Blood Electrification, Brain-Tuner
- Kneeling Bench and LaJiin Bench + Paida Paddle
- SomaVeda® QSRS: Personalized Biophotonics-EMF Protection (SomaVeda® Lifecard™)
- PureWave® and GX9 Vibratory Endermatherpie
- AUTOCONDENSATION, GROUNDING, ELECTRIC CELLULAR MASSAGE: Tesla-Lakhovsky HF, Rife Frequency Generator
- Aroma-Steam
- Bio-Magnetic Therapy: Static Pole Bio-Magnets
- Acu-Spark or similar Piezo-electric point stimulation
- MaGrain Magnetic Pellets for Auricular Acupoint application
- SanMar Rocking Machine ("Chi Machine")
- Miscellaneous "Tok Sen" and Traditional Thai and Ayurveda hand tools for hitting, scraping, and pressure
- Chinese Cupping tools
- *(Note: This list is not exhaustive and is subject to change at any time.)*

51) Bonus! All that there is!

Fifty-two is a metaphor for all the novel possible expressions of this most generous and creatively expressed art and science. Forty-nine is an expression without limitation. Indigenous Traditional Natural Medicine, as an expression of Religious Therapeutics, is an elegant and rich source for healing methodologies.

We stand on the shoulders of giants, drawing on the sophistication and practicality our elders have given us. However, we were given the mandate to ensure our traditional medicine is appropriate for both the people we minister to and the environment in which they live. Environment does not just mean natural surroundings, as it encompasses the entirety of life expression and the surrounding forces that may contribute to separating us from our true nature, our sublime and self-realized consciousness.

Modern science and clinical research may reveal additional systematic approaches to using or emphasizing ITTM. Research and articles on ITTM may be found at. www.ThaiMassage.Com.

This means we are not done. We are developing new and innovative protocols and ministry therapeutics that are cogent with our sacred beliefs and appropriate for the modern conditions of life and society.

What kind of healing system is SomaVeda® to you?

What SomaVeda® Integrated Traditional Therapies®: Indigenous Traditional Thai Yoga is Not!

Very Important! When I wrote and published my first class workbook and eventual textbook ("Nuat Thai, Traditional Thai Medical Massage", Meta Journal Press, Atlanta, GA) in 1983, in the USA, Thailand, Canada, and most of the world, there was no such thing as "Massage Law" or "Massage Therapy Boards" or any variation thereof. Now these kinds of legislative, governmental attempts to control indigenous, traditional, natural medicine from a secular, governmental point of view are becoming quite common.

Due to the expansion of regulation, which primarily seeks to control the use of terms for marketing and taxation under the guise of public safety, the terms "Massage" and "Massage Therapy" have become legally defined as basically "rubbing on the public for money," i.e. Gliding, Stroking, stroking, Thumb press, and Percussion in infinite variation for hire.

The practice of "Massage" is allegedly derived from practices taught and refined by a Swedish gentleman, Per Henrick Ling, in Stockholm around the turn of the century, and was brought to America as a livelihood by Swedish and European immigrants. This mechanical art, defined as an art of physical manipulation, primarily because of its market and financial potential, has become the mainstream's idea of what basic manipulative therapy is in the West.

SomaVeda® ITTM is NOT based on manipulation and never was historically. It was and is a Religious Therapy based on Indigenous Ayurveda, Buddhist Medicine, and other Indigenous traditional medicine practices, addressing suffering caused by separation from knowledge and relationship with God and Spirit.

It is a sad thing that more Vedic and Yoga practitioners, as well as many other legitimate and traditional healing practices, do not define their practices as religious and or religious therapeutics as appropriate. Because of individuals and even some quite large Yoga organizations defining their practices as mere exercise, akin to calisthenics and/or physical manipulation, there is confusion among the public, the lay population, and government agencies.

It is also a sad thing that so many so-called Yoga, Ayurveda, and Yoga Therapy teachers apparently do not know that these practices have always been religious in origin and have always been first and foremost religious therapeutics historically. The known historical figures we claim as our founders have always been referred to as "Saints", "Sages", "Reishi", etc.

Historically, it has been a crime to consider these ancient spiritual people separate and apart from their lifelong devotion to their religious life. They themselves made no bones about it. The purpose of their devotions, their healing practices, their teaching, and their life lived by example was the firmly and deeply held convictions. The ancients believed that these practices provided saving graces, reduced and/or eliminated harmful and obstructive Karma, and removed impediments to becoming enlightened, self-realized conscious beings with truth and transcendent consciousness evident in every thought, action, deed, and word.

They PRAYED for the reduction of suffering for themselves and for the world according to the doctrine, dogma, and contemporary practices of their faith. And yes, they had faith. They had beliefs and firmly held convictions in the unseen.

It does not matter whether they were Hindu, Buddhist, or of another sect. It does not matter whether they were indigenous and or tribal in origin or by association. The body of work, ministry, and methodologies were all focused on singular ends: religious ends and religious-philosophical ends, as are ours.

I will say it once more for emphasis. Just because there are those who, for whatever reason, decide to practice elements of our traditional, indignous and religious therapies for other reasons does not mean that we do not have the right and obligation to continue our traditional practices. Just because the non-religious choose to use the traditional names for what we do does not deprive us, the indigenous and traditional religious practitioners, of the right to practice our faith and the expressions of our faith as they have been responsibly passed down to us.

SomaVeda® ITTM is NOT Massage Therapy nor Massage as defined by most secular state laws in the US. It is not related to or a derivative of Swedish Massage. It is an ancient, indigenous, traditional cultural heritage of the Indigenous Thai people, which has been adopted as a religious therapeutic practice of the Native American Indigenous Church (NAIC) in the US. It is an art which is based on Indigenous Ayurveda, Buddhist, Native American, and Christian principles, as well as the spiritualist beliefs and practices of indigenous, tribal people.

It is news to many uninformed persons that Indigenous, Native Americans can add, incorporate, and practice indigenous, traditional healing, religious therapeutics from any indigenous people found anywhere in the world! Native Americans have been forced to consider Indigenous, traditional healing ways and practices from other aboriginal and indigenous peoples as a result of attrition from the cultural genocide carried out on them, wholesale, for over 100 years in the US. In the past, Medicine Men and Women and their families were actually targeted for atrocity.

As we lost these elders, and/or were prohibited from passing on to the children and tribal communities their medicine knowledge, we lost the ability to practice our religious beliefs, in which medicine, healing practice, and expression were paramount. Under both the US federal code (US Code AIRFA/RLUIPA & Title 18), we are given the right to self-determination and freedom of expression in our religious beliefs and practices. Additionally, under international and UN Human Rights treaties, we are free to determine what these beliefs, practices, and expressions are!

ITTM is not the same as "Massage," "Massage Therapy," or "bodywork," as commonly defined in so-called "Massage Laws." The term “Thai Massage” is Western slang, mostly promoted by tourists in Thailand. Although the term is now common, it is still misunderstood and misused by the misinformed. It is easy to be confused when similar words are used, such as “Massage,” but legally, there are distinctions and differences in definitions.

Please note: In common English, when we, as ITTM practitioners, use the word “massage,” we do not mean it in the same context as the typical Western usage. In the West, “Massage” is often used to mean a “rub down” for money and primarily refers to systems derived from Swedish Massage and Massage Therapy. “ITTM/ Thai Yoga and or Traditional Thai Massage” (*Ráksãa Thaang Nûat Phaen Boran Thai*) is completely unrelated!

Legally, words can have different meanings than in common, non-legal language. For example, the definitions of “massage " and Massage Therapy” are based on the commercial practice of “Swedish massage.” “Swedish Massage” is new (less than one hundred years old) in European and American culture, and it is defined legally as “the application of a system of structured touch, pressure, movement, and holding to the soft tissues of the human body to affect the health and well-being of the client positively. The practice includes the external application of water, heat, cold, lubricants, salt scrubs, and other topical preparations and devices that mimic or enhance the actions of the hands.”

ITTM is a comprehensive, sophisticated healing arts derivative of Theraveda Buddhism, Buddhist medicine, Buddhist Psychology, Theraveda Vipassana Bhavana, Classical Indian and Tibetan Ayurveda, and Yoga Vedanta.

ITTM (Indigenous Traditional Thai Massage/Traditional Thai Yoga) sounds, and in some expressions looks, externally similar to Western-style massage at first glance, but what is not mentioned in the preceding statements is that ITTM is a spiritually based system of healing and movement education (Indigenous, traditional Ayurveda/Yoga). It is based entirely on principles of energy balancing (Sen, Tri-Dosha, Lom, Chakra, etc.), and the actual touching, contact, or soft-tissue manipulation is incidental to, and not the central aim of, the practice!

I want to emphasize this statement again: “It is possible to have an ITTM session with little or no actual touching”. However, touching is good! This work brings fundamental elements and energies into harmony and creates wholeness of mind, body, and spirit (Somatic Homeostasis).

ITTM is a spiritually based Somatic technique and profession, a modality whose standards were established in Buddhist holistic centers and temples thousands of years ago. It has an established code of ethics known as the Buddha Dharma, the Eightfold Path, Ahimsa (non-violence), and the "Ten Rules of the Healer." There is an established criterion for education and professional practice for services that were never intended to be "Massage" or "Massage therapy."

ITTM is founded on spiritual, energetic, and natural principles. These philosophies require practitioners and recipients to profess belief in and to work from a belief in the unseen: Spirit, Puja, Prana (breath of life), Energy, Lom/ Marma, Kwan (consciousness, entity or spirit), Elements Lom: Air, Fai: Fire, Din: Earth and Naam: Water), Humors, and intelligent agencies such as the inherited healing essence and conscious guidance from deceased ancestors and teachers (lineage, Wai Khruu).

Traditional emphasis includes addressing Kwan through rituals such as prayers, mantras, smudging, burning therapeutic and/or blessed Joss (incense), and invoking a deity. Religious and/or spiritual ritual was more common when a malicious agency or Pii (Ghost or Evil Spirit) was considered or diagnosed as causative. This is a very similar concept to that shared in Ayurveda, Chinese medicine, and Native American Medicine: that illness and infirmity can be caused by malicious, pernicious, and/or evil agency that needs to be appeased and/or dispelled by magical practices and incantation (Mantra recitation).

For example, compare traditional Chinese medicine concepts of pathogenesis, citing Pernicious or "Six Evil Influences" as the origin of a disease condition (Classic Chinese Medical Text: Nan Jing). This traditional ritualistic emphasis on belief in the unseen as a common and necessary part of traditional Thai medicine practice was documented by Brun and Schumacher in their seminal work, "Traditional Herbal Medicine in Northern Thailand" (1994 edition, White Lotus, Bangkok, Thailand).

ITTM is a spiritually based system of healing, Religious Therapeutics, Chirothesia, and Somatic therapy in which the healer, practitioner, therapist, or doctor literally becomes the extension of sacred, divine intention and manifestation. It is a direct, literal, practical expression of loving-kindness and compassion, reducing suffering and bringing wellness and happiness to all who are touched by it.

The fact of its apparent sophistication, elegance, efficiency, power, and vitality does not make it merely or simply a system of mechanical manipulation!

For more information on these cultural, religious and legal distinctions presented in this book, see other SomaVeda® textbooks and educational media at https://BeardedMedia.com

ISBN-13: 978-1-886338-52-4

9 781886 338524

53499

Made in United States
Orlando, FL
04 November 2026

90200999R00046